Thrombosis

YOUR PERSONAL HEALTH SERIES

Thrombosis

EVERYTHING YOU NEED TO KNOW

JACK HIRSH, CM, MD, FRCP(C), FRACP, FRSC, DSc

FIREFLY BOOKS

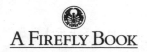

A FIREFLY BOOK

Published by Firefly Books (U.S.) Inc. 2005

First printing

Publisher Cataloging-in-Publication Data (U.S.)

Hirsh, Jack.
   Thrombosis / Jack Hirsh.
[200] p. : ill. ; cm. (Your personal health)
Includes bibliographical references and index.
Summary: Practical health guide to thrombosis for both patients and their families, including advice on diagnosis, treatment options and symptoms.
ISBN 1-55407-096-1 (pbk.)
1. Thrombosis. 2. Thrombolytic therapy. 3. Coronary heart disease. I. Title.
II. Series.
616.1/23 dc22 RC685.C6H577 2005

Published in the United States by
Firefly Books (U.S.) Inc.
P.O. Box 1338, Ellicott Station
Buffalo, New York 14205

Printed in Canada

Acknowledgments

I am grateful for the help of the following people: Jenny Wang wrote the first draft of the section on pediatric thrombosis, reviewed early drafts, and provided valuable comments; Dr. William Geerts reviewed the manuscript extensively and made valuable comments. Drs. Jeff Weitz, Shannon Bates, and Clive Kearon reviewed sections of the manuscript.

Contents

Introduction / 1

Chapter One: Blood in Circulation / 5

Chapter Two: Blood Clots: A Modern Risk for Modern Times / 13

Chapter Three: The Symptoms of Venous Clots / 30

Chapter Four: Diagnosis of Venous Clots / 50

Chapter Five: Prevention of Clots in Veins and Lung Arteries / 59

Chapter Six: Treatment / 65

Chapter Seven: Inherited Thrombophilia / 120

Chapter Eight: Thrombosis in Children / 128

Conclusion / 133

Table of Drug Names / 135

Glossary / 136

Further Resources / 142

Index / 143

Introduction

Normally, blood flows through our arteries and veins smoothly and efficiently, and we never think much about it. However, if a clot blocks the smooth flow of blood, the result can be serious and can even cause death. Diseases arising from clots in blood vessels include heart attacks, stroke and deep venous thrombosis, and pulmonary embolism. These disorders collectively are the commonest cause of death and disability in the developed world. This book is about clots in veins, which cause deep vein thrombosis and pulmonary embolism, as opposed to clots in arteries, which cause heart attacks and stroke. Except in rare circumstances, clots in veins and clots in arteries are caused by different types of disorders, are treated differently, and produce quite different complications.

Many people who develop deep vein thrombosis or pulmonary embolism are anxious because they don't know what to expect in the early stages of their illness (will they get better or not?), what they can and should not do when discharged from hospital while taking oral blood-thinning medication, and what will happen when they stop treatment.

Discontinuing treatment can be especially stressful because at that time people with a history of such clots will be told that they have a risk of developing another episode of clotting or, if their legs are swollen, that the swelling might never go away. Consequently, while they want to be able to recognize the symptoms of a new episode of clotting so that they can go to a hospital emergency room for diagnosis and treatment, they do not want to become neurotic and alarmed by every twinge or ache. For some patients, the fear of another event or the presence of life-long symptoms, such as swelling in the affected leg, looms as a constant reminder of their clotting disorder— rather like a toothache or headache that won't go away and prevents them from enjoying life.

There is no need for pessimism, however, because in most cases the news is good. Many people recover completely and have no further problems from clotting and, in almost all cases, serious complications can be prevented by modern treatments. People with vein clots can play golf, swim, jog, and participate in most activities, even while on blood thinners, and can usually participate in all activities after they have discontinued treatment.

The aim of this book is to allay anxiety and encourage people with clots to live full, normal lives by providing them with information about the symptoms of vein clots, the methods used to diagnose them, the various treatment options, and the risk of complications—both from the treatment they receive and from the vein clots themselves.

As a physician who has been looking after patients with deep vein thrombosis and pulmonary embolism for more than thirty-five years, I never cease to be amazed at how simple answers to my patients' questions provide them with so much relief. When I see a patient for the first time, she or he is often armed with a list of questions and is anxious. Thanks to excellent clinical research in the field of venous thrombosis, most questions can be answered, and patients leave the clinic relieved and with a new resolve. It is my hope that this book will be a convenient and useful source of reference and, by presenting key information, provide relief for the anxious patient, relative, or partner.

Early discoveries

Our modern understanding of the circulation of the blood and the role of the heart as a pump comes from the great discoveries made by William Harvey, a British physician. In the early 1600s, medical experts thought that food was converted to venous blood in the liver and that arterial blood originated from the heart. Harvey thought otherwise and performed experiments that convinced him that blood was pumped from the heart, to which it returned and then recirculated. He also showed that the valves in the veins always directed blood back to the heart. He predicted that the arterial and venous circulations were connected by tiny blood vessels, but it was some years later before the capillaries were observed directly under a microscope.

During the course of a lifetime about one in twenty people will develop a blood clot in their veins, usually in their legs, that will cause discomfort. The discomfort usually takes the form of pain and swelling in the affected leg. The clot can also break off and travel through the bloodstream into the arteries of the lungs and cause chest pain and difficulties with breathing. The medical term for a clot in the vein is "venous thrombosis"; and for clots that develop in deep veins, "deep vein thrombosis." The medical term for a clot that begins in veins and breaks off and travels to the lung is "pulmonary embolism."

About 50 percent of those who develop these kinds of clots will have some other condition that increases their risk, such as a bout with cancer, recent surgery, a serious medical illness, or a serious accident, but for the other 50 percent, the clot can occur "out of the blue." We now know that some people who develop vein clots without obvious cause have an abnormality in their blood that is often inherited.

Most episodes of leg clots are not dangerous, and might not even cause symptoms, but some can be serious; if the clots are large and break off and travel to the lungs they can even cause death. Fortunately, these serious events can usually be prevented by using relatively simple and well proven measures in people who are at risk for venous clotting (for example, those requiring surgery) or by recognizing less serious early signs of leg or lung clots, and treating them promptly.

This book is written for people who, for a number of reasons, have a special interest in blood clots in the veins or lung arteries, perhaps because they:

- suffer from this disorder
- have a relative or friend who has venous thrombosis or pulmonary embolism
- have a family history of blood clots
- are concerned about developing blood clots after exposure to risky situations, such as surgery, major trauma, or long-distance travel
- are concerned about the risk of clots associated with taking estrogen-containing birth control pills or hormone replacement therapy

This book will answer some of the questions that have been asked of me by patients and their physicians during thirty years of supervising a referral clinic for people with suspected venous thrombosis or pulmonary embolism. My goal is to provide the reader with an understanding of the nature of these clots in the legs and lungs; their causes and complications, including post-thrombotic syndrome and pulmonary hypertension; and the methods used to diagnose, prevent, and treat them.

Some of the more difficult concepts are discussed more than once, the repetition reflecting my experience with people who, as they acquire information, often return to questions on some of the more complex topics.

Blood in Circulation

Before we start our discussion of clots in the veins and lung arteries, it is useful to review the way blood circulates through the body under normal circumstances, and how a blood clot can interfere with that circulation.

Blood is pumped through the blood vessels of our body by the heart. The heart pump is a muscle the size of a fist, with left- and right-sided chambers or compartments. Each side consists of an atrium and a ventricle. The atria and ventricles are guarded by valves that ensure that when the chambers contract, blood passes from the atria to the ventricles and from the ventricles to the large arteries of the body. Except in rare circumstances, the left and right chambers are completely separated from each other by a wall of heart muscle known as a septum. The heart chambers contract and relax rhythmically at a rate of about 70 beats per minute. During contraction, blood squirts out of the chambers and during relaxation the chambers refill with blood.

With each contraction, blood is pumped out of the ventricles into a large artery. Blood from the left ventricle is pumped into the aorta and blood from the right ventricle is pumped into the main pulmonary artery. Blood pumped into the aorta transports oxygen and nutrients to the tissues and organs of the body. The aorta branches and divides into smaller arteries, like branches of a tree, that taper down to a vast network of microscopic thin vessels called capillaries. It is here that the oxygen and nutrients are released into the tissues, and are replaced by carbon dioxide and waste products.

Normal Circulation

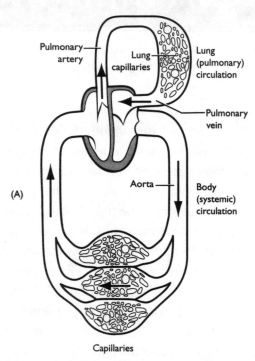

This illustration shows a frontal view of the heart and lungs. After returning to the right side of heart (A), the blood poor in oxygen is pumped into the pulmonary arteries for transportation to the lungs where it receives oxygen from the air that we breathe and then returns the oxygenated blood to the left side of the heart.

The capillaries from the systemic circulation then join up again to form a network of veins that transport the blood back to the right side of the heart. There, the nonoxygenated blood, now a dark bluish-red, is pumped into the arteries of the lungs (pulmonary arteries) where it travels to the lung's capillaries. While in the lungs, the blood picks up oxygen from the air that we inhale and the carbon dioxide is released into the lungs (and eventually exhaled). The oxygen-containing blood, now bright red (because of the oxygen) re-enters the left side of the heart through the pulmonary veins for another cycle through the body.

Thus, there are two main circulatory systems: systemic circulation, through which the blood transports life-giving oxygen and nutrients to the body and removes waste products for disposal; and the pulmonary circulation that transports the oxygen-depleted blood from the right side of the heart to the lungs, where the blood is replenished with oxygen, and then returned to the heart. These two circulations are separated by walls inside the heart, and the tiny microscopic capillaries in the lungs prevent clots that form in the veins from passing into the systemic circulation.

People who develop blood clots in veins are sometimes concerned that the clot might cause a heart attack or stroke. There is no need to be anxious, since the fine capillary network in the lungs acts as a filter that prevents clots that form in veins from passing into the systemic circulation (and therefore into the arteries that supply the heart or brain); thus, people with clots in veins can be reassured that these types of clots don't cause heart attacks or stroke.

Blood Clotting in Arteries and Veins

Under normal circumstances, blood remains fluid because both the inner lining of the blood vessels (called the endothelium) and the blood contain substances that prevent it from clotting. If a blood vessel is cut (for example, as a result of injury, surgery, or childbirth), blood flows out of the vessel where it comes in contact with very powerful substances contained in the tissues in and around the vessel wall that stimulate blood clotting and seal the leak. The seal, known as a hemostatic plug, is made up of clumps of sticky particles, called blood platelets, and congealed blood.

The hemostatic plug forms a scab that hardens and then disappears over a period of days or weeks, during which time the blood vessel is repaired. This process—hemostatic plug formation followed by a scab—is similar to what happens to an external cut.

Venous Clot Formation

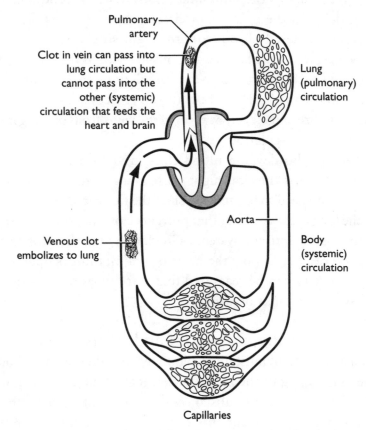

A clot in a vein can pass into lung circulation but cannot pass into the other (systemic) circulation that feeds the heart, brain, and other organs.

A clot in a lung (pulmonary) artery is prevented from passing into the body (systemic) arterial circulation by the pulmonary capillaries.

This type of beneficial clotting is a vital protective mechanism without which we would bleed to death. However, when clots form *inside* blood vessels, where they can interfere with normal blood flow, they can be harmful. The medical term for this kind of clot is thrombus, or thrombosis. Such clots are a relatively recent development in human evolution, and may have been brought about by changes in our diet and life-style and by improvements in medical technology that have prolonged our lives (e.g., intensive care units, anesthesia, transplantation, cancer treatments, etc.). This book focuses on these harmful clots when they affect veins and lungs.

Blood clots are made up of a mesh of strands called fibrin, along with the small sticky particles called blood platelets. Other blood cells are trapped in the clot but are not actively involved in the clotting process. The clots can obstruct blood flow in the vessel, or they can break off and follow the flow of the blood upstream. A clot that breaks off in this way is called an embolism. When a clot forms in a vein or artery, a number of things can happen to it. The clot can grow and continue to block the vessel either partly or completely; it might shrink and leave a scar; or it can be dissolved by the body's natural clot-dissolving systems and disappear completely without leaving a scar.

Treatment of a clot with blood-thinning drugs, called anti-thrombotic or anticoagulant drugs, reduces the risk that the clot will grow and allows the body's natural system to remove it. Treatment with clot-dissolving drugs, called fibrinolytic agents (or clot-busters), speeds up the disappearance or disso-lution of the clot.

Arterial Clots

When clots form in arteries the consequences are generally more serious than when they form in veins, because arteries carry life-giving oxygenated blood and nutrients from the heart chambers to the heart muscle, brain, kidneys, and other vital organs. A clot in an artery can interrupt blood flow to these major organs.

To the Heart

For example, if the clot completely blocks an artery that supplies the heart, heart tissue begins to die in minutes. After six to twelve hours the damage is permanent, resulting in a heart attack (myocardial infarction). If the blockage is partial, the person can suffer a minor attack or just have severe chest pain without any permanent damage to the heart muscle (so-called unstable angina).

Arterial Blood Clots

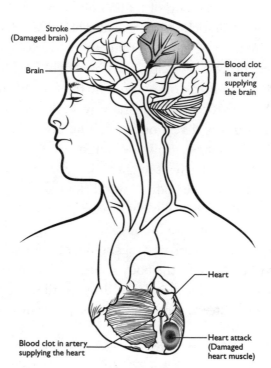

This illustration shows a clot in the coronary artery (supplying the heart muscle). The clot causes a blockage, which in turn leads to a heart attack and a clot in a cerebral artery (supplying the brain) that has caused a stroke.

To the Brain

If the clot forms in an artery supplying oxygen to the brain, it can cause a stroke. The brain tissue fed by these arteries will be damaged within minutes and will be permanently damaged within approximately three hours.

To the Legs

If the clot forms in the arteries supplying the legs, it can cause gangrene of the affected leg. Gangrene means dead tissue. A gangrenous leg looks black and is treated by amputation.

Venous Clots

Blood moving through arteries is traveling at great speeds and under high pressure. In contrast, blood flows through the venous system much more slowly and under much lower pressure. Blood clots that obstruct veins are usually less serious than arterial clots. If a vein is completely blocked, the blood can return to the heart through alternate venous channels. These venous clots only very, very rarely cause the tissues of the leg to die. However a venous clot can break off and result in a pulmonary embolism. Most pulmonary embolisms are not fatal and, as already discussed, clots in veins do not cause heart attacks or stroke because they are prevented from passing into the systemic circulation (and therefore into the arteries of the heart and brain) by the tiny capillaries in the lung.

About one in twenty people in North America and Europe will develop a venous clot or lung embolism in their lifetime, most occurring in those 40 years of age or older. Venous clots develop when the normal processes that function to keep blood fluid are disturbed. Blood can be stimulated to clot if either the inner lining of the vein is damaged, or if substances that trigger clotting are released into the blood.

The chances of developing a significant venous clot when the clotting process is stimulated are increased if the blood is allowed to pool in the legs, for example, during periods of prolonged bed rest or sitting in a cramped position, or if a person has an inherited genetic defect in certain anticlotting proteins that counteract the blood's tendency to clot. These processes that lead to clot formation are discussed in more detail in the next chapter.

Normal Valve Function

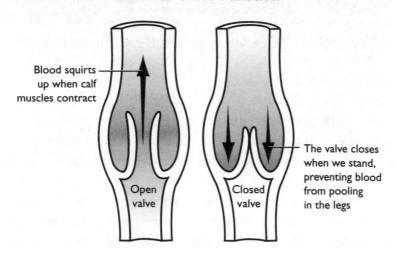

Blood squirts up when calf muscles contract

Open valve

Closed valve

The valve closes when we stand, preventing blood from pooling in the legs

Because the venous circulation is a low-pressure system, veins have a series of valves that ensure that blood moves in one direction, back to the heart. If it were not for these valves, blood would pool in our legs when we stand for prolonged periods, and lead to leg swelling. When we walk and contract our leg muscles, the blood is squeezed up toward the heart and when we stand still, the venous valves prevent blood from pooling in the legs. Most venous thrombi are thought to start in the valve pockets in the veins of the calf, because it is here that blood tends to stagnate, particularly during periods of inactivity.

TWO

Blood Clots: A Modern Risk for Modern Times

Scientific studies suggest that prior to the twentieth century, venous clotting was very rare. Today, this condition affects one in twenty people in the Western world during the course of their lifetime. Consequently, there are millions of people throughout the Western world who have suffered or will suffer from blood clots in their leg veins. Most of these people are over 40, and many are over 60, but clots can also occur in young people.

Who Is at Risk?

Given that many of the risks associated with increased venous clotting are a product of our modern society, you would expect this condition to be much less common in developing countries, and this is the case. In Western countries about 1 in 1,000 people develop venous clots every year. This translates into about 5 percent of the population, or 1 in 20 in a lifetime. In Africa and certain parts of Asia, the risk is much lower (a tenth or less of the risk in Westerners).

In general, we divide risk factors into those that are temporary, such as surgery, and those that are permanent, such as age and genetics. There is a further distinction—namely whether or not the risk factors can be changed. For example, obesity and the use of estrogens are risk factors that can be altered, but genetics cannot yet.

Some of the common risk factors have already been described; however, not all clots occur in association with obvious risk factors. Some blood clots occur without prior warning and some people with such clots have a blood abnormality that increases their risk of clotting. These blood abnormalities are often inherited.

Risk Factors

The reason that such a large number of people develop clots lies in the technological developments that have occurred during the last century, increasing the number of people who have one of several risk factors that we now know promote clotting. The common risk factors include:

- major surgery
- severe accidental trauma (for example, from motor vehicle accidents)
- prolonged bed rest due to illness
- chronic debilitating illnesses
- leg paralysis
- cancer
- old age
- estrogens
- previous venous thrombosis

Major surgery, for example, with its requirement for anesthesia and intensive care units, has been possible for less than a century. Until very recently people with serious illnesses were not kept alive in our intensive care units, women did not take estrogens, and people with cancer did not survive long enough to develop a clot. Nowadays, people exercise less, are more obese, and live much longer. All of these factors and certain other accompaniments of modern living increase the frequency and likelihood of developing venous clots.

However, not all clots occur in association with obvious risk factors. Some blood clots occur spontaneously, without prior warning, and some people with such clots have a blood abnormality that increases their risk of clotting. These blood abnormalities are often inherited.

The risk factors listed above promote clotting in one or more of four ways by:

- releasing pro-clotting chemicals into the blood
- failing to block these clot-promoting factors
- causing damage to veins
- interfering with the free circulation of blood, causing blood to stagnate in the veins of the legs

Let's consider these four ways of stimulating clot formation in more detail.

- Clot-promoting factors result in the production of an enzyme called *thrombin* that converts fluid blood into a solid mass, the blood clot. This process of blood clotting—which occurs when the body is injured or tissues are damaged—seals blood vessels and thereby stems the flow of blood when a blood vessel is cut. It is a vital process that is present in the animal kingdom and has evolved over millions of years.

- The body has also developed a system that regulates thrombin formation and confines its action to the site of the cut blood vessel. This system prevents excessive clotting. Sometimes people are born with a defect in their natural *anticoagulant* system (due to a genetic mutation). This is called *thrombophilia*, which means a tendency to form clots, the opposite of *hemophilia*, which is a tendency to bleed excessively.
- When a vein is damaged, very small clots form as part of the healing process. If there are defects in the normal checks and balances that accompany this process, these very small clots can grow and cause problems by blocking blood flow.
- Free-flowing blood in veins prevents clotting by washing away clot-inducing substances, such as thrombin, and by breaking up small clots that form at the site of blood vessel damage, thereby preventing them from growing into large clots. When people are confined to bed and don't or can't move their legs, blood stagnates (or pools) in the leg veins and the protection afforded by flowing blood is lost.

Let's now consider the common risk factors for venous clots in more detail.

Major Surgery and Major Trauma

Major surgery and trauma result in the release of chemicals into the circulation that increase clotting and prevent the clot from being dissolved. Nature has designed our system to minimize bleeding in response to trauma by speeding up the clotting process and by strengthening the clot. This makes perfect sense because, prior to modern times, man's greatest threat to life was uncontrollable bleeding from injury (for example, during battle or when attacked by wild animals). Now the human race is confronted by a different threat, the threat of thrombosis. Bleeding during injury from surgery or motor vehicle accidents can now be controlled and rarely causes death. However, when exposed to injury, the body is still programmed to produce substances to slow bleeding. It has therefore unwittingly turned this life-saving protective process into a dangerous one that can promote vein clots. Either surgery or trauma to the legs and pelvis can also injure veins. Major surgery is associated with enforced immobility during anesthetic and while the person is recovering, thereby promoting the pooling of blood in the leg veins. Therefore, major surgery and serious trauma is associated with all four factors that promote clots in veins. Fortunately we can anticipate and prevent this problem by using well-developed preventative measures.

Cancer

Cancer predisposes people to venous clotting in a number of ways. In people who have advanced cancers, clot-promoting chemicals are released into the bloodstream both by the cancer cells themselves and as a result of chemotherapy or radiotherapy, the treatments for cancer. These cancer treatments injure normal cells as well as cancer cells, both of which release clot-promoting substances into the blood. Cancer patients are often immobile as well, encouraging the pooling of blood in the veins of the legs.

Less commonly, venous clots are the first signs of undetected cancer in an otherwise symptom-free person. It should be stressed that most people with venous clots neither have nor will develop cancer, but in a small percentage, cancer that is undetectable when a person seeks medical attention for vein clots will become evident within the next two years. It's thought that these patients already have microscopic nests of cancer cells in their system, and that even these few cancer cells are producing the powerful clot-promoting factors that are later seen in more advanced cancers.

Common Risk Factors for Venous Clots

Risk factor	Increase blood clotting	Damage veins	Pooling of blood in legs
Major surgery*	++++	++	++++
Major trauma to legs and pelvis*	++++	++++	++++
Prolonged bed rest and immobility*	–	++	++++
Cancer*	++++	–	++
Age*	+		+++
Family predisposition*	++++	–	–
Previous venous thrombosis*	++	–	+
Estrogens	++	–	+
Pregnancy	++		+
Heart failure	–	–	++++
Chronic illness	++	–	++
Varicose veins	–	++	++++
Obesity	+	–	++

*major risk factors

The number of + signs indicate the strength of the association between the clinical risk factor and the causes of clotting.

In those people with venous clots who are otherwise well, the risk of subsequently developing cancer in the following two years is about one in thirty. If other features of illness are present when the person experiences these blood clots—such as weight loss or anemia—then the chance that a cancer will show up in the next six to twelve months is higher.

The possibility of having an associated cancer (among people who present with vein clots without any obvious cause) has led some doctors to suggest that such patients should be investigated for the possible presence of cancer. However, whether or not doctors should pursue this kind of testing is controversial. At our institution, we investigate people who present with venous clots for cancer only if they have other features of the illness, such as weight loss or unexplained anemia (low blood count), for example. We have found that a comprehensive search for cancer in a person with venous clots who is otherwise well is generally not fruitful, as falsely positive tests can lead to a chain of events that are not only frustrating to the patient, but also can cause harm. If you have a blood clot, your doctor will be able to discuss this issue with you and decide whether further testing is necessary or not.

Age

Increasing age is also an important risk factor. For people between 15 and 30 years of age, for example, the baseline risk of venous thrombosis is about 1 in 10,000 per year. In contrast, for those over 80 the risk is about 1 in 100 per year. The reason for this increasing risk as we age is due in part to the frequent presence of associated illness, the need for surgery, and an increased frequency of cancer. However, with age, it is also likely that the blood vessels' lining loses some of the properties that protect them against clotting, and the veins of the leg lose their tone, leading to an increased probability of the pooling of stagnant blood and clot formation.

Inherited Thrombophilia

A significant number of people under the age of 50 who go to their doctors with vein clots or clots in their lung, but without other major risk factors, have an inherited or genetic protein abnormality that predisposes them or other members of their family to venous clots. As already mentioned, this condition is known as inherited thrombophilia (see Chapter Seven for a more thorough discussion of this topic).

To date, five proven inherited clotting disorders have been identified. The various disorders result from mutations in the genes responsible for making five different anticlotting proteins:

- antithrombin
- protein C

- protein S
- Factor V (known as Factor V Leiden)
- prothrombin

Collectively, these conditions are called inherited thrombophilia. The Factor V Leiden mutation is the most common, occurring in one in twenty otherwise normal people in Western populations. The prothrombin mutation occurs in about one in fifty, and the other three are much less common. People who inherit these defective proteins have an increased risk for venous clots.

Not every member of a family affected by one of these mutations is at increased risk for thrombosis. On average, about 50 percent of family members will carry these genetic mutations. But most individuals with an abnormal protein will not develop thrombosis in their lifetime.

The chances that an asymptomatic carrier (a family member with one of these genetic mutations) of one of these familial thrombophilic disorders will develop a venous clot depends on the disorder. The risk is increased about twofold with the prothrombin mutation, four- to fivefold with the Factor V Leiden mutation, and about ten- to twentyfold with each of the other three conditions: deficiencies of protein C, protein S, and antithrombin. These increased risks translate into an increased lifetime risk of venous thrombosis. As discussed, the lifetime risk of venous thrombosis in a person without thrombophilia is 5 percent; that is, about one in twenty people without one of these conditions will develop venous clots during their lifetime, usually after the age of 40, and more often after the age of 60. In contrast, the lifetime risk of venous clotting for a person with the Factor V Leiden mutation is about 20 percent, or one in five. The lifetime risk associated with deficiencies in antithrombin, protein C, or protein S is even higher. People with inherited thrombophilia often develop thrombosis at a young age. Therefore, inherited thrombophilia should be suspected if a number of people in the family have venous clots or if a person develops a venous clot before the age of 40. Inherited thrombophilia is not a risk factor for heart attacks or stroke.

Still, even though these individuals are at increased risk for venous clots, it is not customary to routinely treat carriers with blood-thinning drugs to prevent clotting because the blood-thinning medications used to prevent these clots carry their own risks, principally by causing bleeding complications. The risk of death associated with these bleeds is higher than that from venous clots in carriers with no symptoms. Therefore, doctors generally limit the use of blood-thinning drugs to high-risk situations, such as when individuals who carry these mutations undergo surgery.

In families with the genetic mutations that cause inherited thrombophilia, about 50 percent of family members will inherit the gene. Those individuals who do not inherit a mutation cannot transmit it to their offspring; you either have or do not have the protein abnormality. However, most people who carry the abnormality do not in fact develop thrombosis in their lifetime. When people find out that they have an inherited thrombophilia, they often become anxious and even depressed. However, there is no need for pessimism. The presence of inherited thrombophilia does not reduce an individual's lifespan—in other words, it does not lead to premature death. When an affected person is exposed to a high-risk situation (such as surgery), many episodes of thrombosis can be prevented by using appropriate preventative measures and, even if thrombosis does occur, it can be readily treated.

When a family member is found to carry one of these abnormalities, other family members often request screening, which is done as much to identify a carrier as it is to give peace of mind to noncarriers. As we discussed previously, people who

The benefits of screening

If, for example, a woman knows that she has familial thrombophilia, she can avoid factors that might compound her increased risk, such as the use of estrogens either for birth control or hormone replacement.

If a familial thrombophilia is found during screening or after a first episode of venous clotting, it could influence the duration of treatment with blood thinners (see Chapter 5, Treatment).

In many cases, screening for familial thrombophilia can be quite helpful. Finally, it is reassuring for other members of the family to know that they do not carry the mutation because they then know that they cannot pass the disorder on to their children. Some people may prefer not to know one way or the other, and that is their choice to make.

have a familial thrombophilia—discovered by routine screening—do not normally receive blood-thinning medication, since their degree of risk does not warrant such treatment. Some authorities advocate against screening for thrombophilia. The case for screening is explained in the sidebar above.

Unlike hemophilia, an inherited condition where males have an increased tendency to bleed, inherited thrombophilia affects both sexes equally. However, the comparison of hemophilia with thrombophilia is useful to consider because hemophilia is caused by genetic mutations in coagulation proteins, that result in delayed blood clotting, causing abnormal bleeding. In contrast, thrombophilia is caused by genetic mutations in proteins that result in a speeding up of the clotting process, predisposing affected people to venous clots.

The first inherited blood abnormality (antithrombin deficiency) was identified about sixty years ago, and the others in the last thirty years. It is likely that there are other as-yet undiscovered abnormalities that lead to abnormal blood clotting and that with further improvements in genetic testing additional inherited thrombophilic defects will be found in people who develop clots without a detectable blood abnormality and without an obvious major risk factor for clotting.

Mrs. C, aged 40, has two teenaged daughters: Ellen and Anna. Mrs. C's maternal uncle died of a pulmonary embolism. Anna was taking a birth control pill, and her mother had read that birth control pills increase the risk of clotting, particularly in women who have a familial clotting disorder. She sought help from her family physician who sent Mrs. C and her two daughters to my clinic for further advice. A complete family history was obtained. Mrs. C did not have a history of venous clots, and neither did her siblings. Her father died of a heart attack and her mother was alive and did not have a history of clotting. Her uncle had developed a pulmonary embolism after hip surgery. Based on this family history it was unlikely that the girls would have a familial clotting disorder (inherited thrombophilia). The pulmonary embolism that developed in her uncle occurred after a well-recognized risk factor, and her father had an arterial thrombosis and not a venous thrombosis.

Mrs. C was told that the chance of finding an inherited clotting disorder in her daughters was no higher than the average person without a family history of a clotting disorder and that the risk was about one in fifteen. Mrs. C remained concerned. Therefore, in order to allay her anxiety, we tested her daughters. The tests were normal, and they were told that the risk of venous clotting was no greater than that which normally occurs with estrogen use.

Since venous thrombosis is a common disorder, it is common to have a family member who has had venous clotting. If at least two family members have a history of venous thrombosis or pulmonary embolism, we would recommend testing for familial thrombophilia in women who are concerned about thrombosis associated with taking estrogen.

Other Blood Abnormalities

Noninherited blood abnormalities can also increase an individual's risk of developing a venous clot. The most important of

Thrombosis and SLE

If a person with thrombosis is found to have a lupus anticoagulant and none of the other features of SLE, he or she can be reassured that it is very unlikely that SLE will develop. SLE is a chronic condition that can cause joint pain and swelling, a rash, a kidney disorder, stroke, and other symptoms. People with SLE do have a higher risk for developing a lupus anticoagulant and for developing blood clots in arteries as well as in veins.

these abnormalities is caused by antiphospholipid antibodies. There are two main types of antiphospholipid antibodies. These are called lupus anticoagulant and anticardiolipin antibodies. Both classes of antibodies can increase the risk of clotting. The term "lupus anticoagulant" is confusing because we would expect the term "anticoagulant" to be associated with bleeding rather than clotting. The lupus anticoagulant was originally described in a patient with the disease systemic lupus erythematosus (SLE). It is now known to occur in many people who do not have SLE. The antibody was shown to interfere with normal clotting in the test tube but was found to be associated with increased clotting in the body. Approximately 2 in 100 unaffected people have the lupus anticoagulant.

Whether or not lupus anticoagulant increases an individual's risk for vein clots depends on the context in which the antibody is found. If it is found in a routine blood screen, there is little need for concern, because it is unlikely to cause thrombosis. In contrast, if a lupus anticoagulant is found in a person who already has a venous clot, it can increase the risk for another bout of thrombosis when anticoagulation therapy, given for the first event, is discontinued. Therefore, the finding of a lupus anticoagulant in association with thrombosis might influence the doctor's decision about how long to continue anticoagulant therapy (see Chapter Six).

Women with antiphospholipid antibodies are also at risk for miscarriage during pregnancy, probably because the antibodies can lead to clotting in the blood vessels supplying the placenta.

Estrogens

Taken either as oral contraception or as hormone replacement therapy after menopause, estrogens are known to increase the risk for clotting by three- to fourfold. The importance of this increased risk depends on each woman's baseline risk. For example, for a woman in good health, with none of the other risk factors for venous clotting that we've discussed, the risk of dying from a blood clot associated with estrogen therapy is much less than the risk of dying in a motor vehicle accident. However, in women with other risk factors, such a history of clotting or an inherited thrombophilia, this three- to fourfold increase in risk could be too dangerous for them to consider using estrogens. For this reason, women who carry one of the inherited thrombophilias or other risk factors for thrombosis are often counseled to be wary of taking estrogens. In these high-risk patients, the underlying risk for venous clotting, together with the three- to fourfold increased risk of clotting from the use of estrogens tips the risk-benefit balance away from estrogen use.

Mrs. B, aged 44, has two daughters: Rita, aged 15, and Sara, aged 17. Her maternal uncle died of a pulmonary embolism, and one of Mrs. B's two brothers developed venous thrombosis at the age of 30 and is on blood thinners. Her mother was thought to have had venous thrombosis during pregnancy. Sara was taking a birth control pill. Mrs. B had read that birth control pills increase the risk of clotting in women who have a familial clotting disorder. She sought help from her family physician who sent Mrs. B and her two daughters to my clinic for further advice. Based on this family history, it was possible that one or both girls would have a familial clotting disorder (inherited thrombophilia). Mrs. B and Rita had a Factor V Leiden defect. Sara was free of any abnormalities and was told that she was not a carrier and would not pass the abnormality on to her children; therefore, there was no reason she could not continue to use the oral contraceptive pill. Mrs. B and Rita were reassured that Factor V Leiden is a common condition and that there was a 75 percent chance that they would not develop venous thrombosis during their lifetime. They were warned that the use of estrogens either for birth control or hormone replacement would increase their risk of thrombosis about threefold and were instructed to ensure that preventative measures be taken if they were ever exposed to a high-risk situation (for example, surgery). The subject of future pregnancy was discussed, and Rita was told that she would not require treatment with blood thinners during pregnancy.

The combination of a Factor V Leiden abnormality and estrogen use increases the risk of venous thrombosis by about fifteenfold. An unaffected female between the ages of 15 and 40 has a risk of thrombosis of 1 in 10,000 per year, whereas the presence of a Factor V abnormality increases this to 1 in 2,000 per year (still very low). The addition of an estrogen-containing compound increases the risk to about 1 in 500 per year, or 1 in 50 over 10 years. If Mrs. B were to consider hormone replacement when she becomes menopausal (as she enters her fifties), the risk of venous thrombosis over a ten-year period would be about one in ten. Therefore, in general, the use of estrogen-containing medication is discouraged in women with Factor V Leiden.

History of Previous Venous Thrombosis

A previous history of a venous clot is also a strong risk factor for the development of a second and third episode. About half of the recurrent episodes occur in the same leg as the initial venous clot, and half occur in the other leg. There are several reasons the occurrence of an initial venous clot increases the risk of a second clot. First, by damaging the vein, the initial clot can interfere with the protective effects of the inner lining of the vein wall. Second, by damaging the valves or obstructing the vein, the initial clot can cause blood to pool in the legs. Finally, in those whose initial clot was caused by a blood abnormality (either detected or undetected), the underlying abnormality will continue to predispose them to further episodes of venous clotting. People who suffer one or more episodes of thrombosis are sometimes treated with blood thinners for an indefinite duration. When they stop blood thinners, they are told to use preventative measures whenever they are exposed to a high-risk situation.

Other Risk Factors

Some chronic illnesses, such as severe inflammatory bowel disease, are associated with an increased risk for venous blood clots. During relapses of this and other illnesses, the risk of clotting is further increased by the immobility that results from being confined to bed. Severe heart disease causing heart failure is also associated with pooling of blood in the leg veins.

Varicose veins are an important risk factor for "superficial" vein clots, that is, clots near the surface of the skin, but are only a weak risk factor for the more important deep vein clots that will be discussed later.

Paralysis of the legs from stroke or spinal cord damage is associated with severe pooling of blood in leg veins and with an increased risk of thrombosis. This risk is highest soon after the stroke or spinal cord injury, because at that time the release of clot-promoting factors from the damaged brain (in the case of stroke) or from the injured tissues associated with the spinal cord damage is coupled with venous blood pooling.

Obesity is a very important risk factor for arterial thrombosis (which causes heart attacks and strokes) and is also associated with an increased risk of venous clots. Obese people's ability to dissolve clots and remain mobile is reduced. Obesity is an important risk factor for venous clotting after surgery.

Smoking is a very important risk factor for heart attacks. It has also recently been shown to be a weak risk factor for venous clots, providing yet another reason to avoid this habit.

Long distance air travel as a risk factor for venous clotting has recently received a great deal of attention in the press, but in fact, it is a very minor risk factor. We now know that the risk is confined almost exclusively to travelers who have other risk factors (see table on page 18), and to flights that take six hours or longer. The risk during one of these lengthy flights is probably increased about threefold over the baseline risk of that person had he or she not traveled. Since the average risk of thrombosis is about 1 in 300,000 per day, an increase to 1 in 100,000 per day in an otherwise healthy traveler is not a serious concern. On the other hand, a threefold increase in risk might be important among those who already have a high risk for clotting.

Two factors are thought to contribute to the increased risk associated with air travel. The first and most important is the risk associated with blood pooling in the legs during prolonged sitting. The second, and of less certain importance, is the dehydration that results from sitting in a pressurized cabin, which can cause blood to thicken, causing sluggish blood flow in the veins. During flight, the skin and breath lose moisture due to the dryness of the cabin air. Drinking alcoholic beverages or coffee during the flight compounds fluid loss, because these beverages contribute to dehydration by promoting urination.

However, because the importance of this suggested cause is uncertain, drinking coffee or alcohol is not prohibited during a long flight, but maintaining good hydration by drinking plenty of water is encouraged.

The risk of venous clotting during long car or bus trips is less well established. Although car travelers are exposed to some of the same risk factors that occur during long flights—prolonged sitting, for example—it is much easier to prevent the pooling of blood in the legs during car or bus travel.

THREE

The Symptoms of Venous Clots

In this and following chapters, case studies will be used to emphasize key points related to the symptoms, diagnosis, prevention and treatment of venous thrombosis and pulmonary embolism.

Venous Thrombosis

Li, aged 65, had an uncomplicated hip replacement operation and was discharged from the hospital to rehabilitate at home. Two weeks later he woke one morning with pain and swelling in his left calf. He tolerated the pain for two days, but it gradually became more severe and he returned to hospital where an ultrasound test showed that he had a large clot in his operated leg. He was treated as an outpatient and made a good recovery.

Hip surgery is an important risk factor for vein clots because it combines immobility, damage to veins (close to the site of surgery), and tissue damage as a result of surgery. In Li's case the symptoms were typical, and he understood he had to return to hospital when his symptoms persisted and was able to receive treatment in a timely manner. He made a very good recovery. If treated early, people with clots in their leg veins typically do very well.

The most common symptoms of venous clots are pain and swelling in the leg. The most common site of pain is the calf, but the pain can start in the groin or even in the buttock. Pain usually precedes swelling, but sometimes both occur together. The pain can be mild or severe, and in some people swelling is the main symptom. It can be confined to the calf or involve the whole leg. The leg can become reddish or purple. Usually, only one leg is affected. The pain, swelling, and discoloration are caused by obstruction or blockage of a major vein or by inflammation of the vein wall. Venous clots produce these symptoms by causing blood to back up below the obstruction, which causes the leg to swell, or by damaging the vein wall and causing it and the surrounding tissues to become inflamed. Sometimes the inflammation is marked and is accompanied by severe pain, redness, and swelling.

Not all venous clots produce marked symptoms. Many clots produce no symptoms, and in some people the symptoms are quite mild—slight calf tenderness or swelling. Although patients with marked symptoms usually have large clots, people can have large clots with mild or even no symptoms in their legs.

If the clot breaks away from the mass formed in the leg and travels to the lungs, the person can develop symptoms of pulmonary embolism. Blood returning through the venous circulation to the right side of the heart normally goes on through to the arteries of the lungs, where it is replenished with oxygen. However, when a clot from the legs is swept along this path with the blood, it can block a lung artery, preventing the blood from taking on oxygen, and cause chest pain and shortness of breath.

The chest pain is usually sharp and aggravated by breathing and coughing. This type of pain, which is known as pleurisy, is caused by inflammation of the membrane (called the pleura) that surrounds the lungs. There are two layers of pleura that are normally separated by a thin layer of fluid. The sharp pleuritic pain occurs because the inflamed membranes rub against each other during breathing or coughing. People with pleuritic chest pain often take rapid shallow breaths to reduce the pain. Less commonly the pain is dull, constant, not aggravated by breathing, and positioned in the center of the chest. Shortness of breath is the most common symptom.

There are two main causes of shortness of breath. The first is related to the pain of breathing caused by the pleuritic pain. The second, which often occurs without pain, is caused by the obstruction to one or more large lung (pulmonary) arteries. Such obstruction interferes with the ability of the lungs to provide adequate amounts of oxygen to blood that normally flows to the lung vessels.

Most people with pulmonary embolism also have clots in their leg veins, but the clots produce symptoms in the legs in only about 30 percent of these patients.

Joan, aged 55, had fallen on the ice and fractured her right ankle. The leg was splinted for six weeks. When her splint was removed she noticed that her right leg was more swollen than the left. She thought that the swelling was a result of the fracture and did nothing about it. However, the swelling did not go away and two weeks later she developed a sharp pain in the right side of her chest and had difficulty breathing. Breathing or coughing made the pain much worse. She tolerated these symptoms for a day and then became very short of breath, felt faint, and collapsed. She was rushed to hospital where examination and tests confirmed the presence of a large blood clot in her right leg and large clots in lung arteries (pulmonary emboli) on both sides. She was admitted to intensive care with a guarded prognosis. Fortunately, she responded to treatment and, after two weeks, recovered enough to be discharged home. She eventually made a complete recovery from the chest pain and shortness of breath; however, even after two years, she still has some leg swelling.

A leg fracture is also a risk factor for clotting in veins because the affected leg is immobilized in a splint for an extended period of time. In this case the mild symptoms gave Joan a false sense of security and she disregarded them. While Joan made a good recovery, she was left with leg swelling because the clot in her vein produced permanent damage to her venous valves. The messages from this example are that very large and dangerous clots can produce minimal symptoms and, with modern treatment, patients can recover from even very large pulmonary emboli.

Fortunately, most venous clots are not dangerous and even if they are large, serious complications can be prevented providing the clots are diagnosed early and treated correctly. Whether or not a venous clot is serious depends on the size of the clot as well as the size and location of the veins that become obstructed. Clots in small veins are less serious than those in large veins. They can become serious if they break off and travel to the lungs. Pulmonary emboli are most dangerous if they are large or if the person is already ill with a weak heart or with lung disease and therefore cannot tolerate even a moderate-sized clot. A small clot that breaks off and travels to the lungs in an otherwise healthy person often causes no symptoms. If Joan had not been a fit person, but instead had been ill with heart or lung disease, the pulmonary embolism might have been fatal.

Venous clots do occur in other veins in the body, but most form in the veins deep within the leg and pelvis rather than superficial veins (those just under the skin's surface). Clots that form in deep veins of the legs or pelvis are known as deep vein thrombosis. Less commonly, though, clots do form in the veins of the arms, and much less commonly, in the veins draining blood from the brain, eyes, intestines, liver, or kidneys. Most of this book is devoted to deep vein thrombosis, but clots in these other venous sites will be examined later.

As already stated, clots in veins do not normally cause heart attacks or strokes because the venous circulation is separated from the arterial circulation by the walls inside the heart and by the capillaries, which are tiny blood vessels in the lung. Rather, it is clots in arteries that normally cause heart attacks and strokes. Very rarely though, patients with a small hole in the wall separating the right side of their heart from the left can suffer a stroke from a vein clot if it slips through the hole (called a *patent foramen ovale*) and passes into the high-pressure arterial circulation, blocking an artery in the brain.

Let's now review the main features of deep vein thrombosis and pulmonary embolism.

Leg Vein Thrombosis

Leg veins can be divided into two groups: the deep veins and the superficial veins. Deep veins are not visible because they are deep in the muscles of the leg. Superficial veins are just under the skin and can be seen easily. The deep veins are divided further into proximal veins (veins above the knee) and calf veins (veins below the knee). In general, clots in calf veins and superficial veins are much smaller than clots in proximal veins. Clots that form in the deep veins above the knee are the most serious: they tend to be large and are therefore more likely to cause leg symptoms. They are also more likely to break off and travel to the lung and result in a pulmonary embolism.

Deep vein thrombosis is sometimes referred to as phlebitis, but in fact these terms have slightly different meanings. Strictly speaking, "phlebitis" is a term used to describe an inflamed vein (usually caused by a venous clot that produces inflammation of the vein wall) while "thrombosis" is a term that refers to a blood clot in a vein or artery. Phlebitis is often used to describe the red, tender, cord-like streak that is characteristic of superficial vein clots, but it can also complicate deep vein clots, resulting in marked redness, pain, and local swelling. The early symptoms of deep venous clots are less severe if they are not accompanied by phlebitis. However, venous clots can sometimes be even more dangerous if they do not produce phlebitis, because the absence of early symptoms can lead to a false sense of security. The following examples illustrate the differences between deep vein thrombosis without and with phlebitis and between deep vein thrombosis and superficial vein thrombosis.

Maya, aged 69, had a gall bladder operation. She recovered from the operation and was discharged home. Two weeks later she developed sharp chest pain and had difficulty breathing. She returned to hospital and a diagnosis of pulmonary embolism was made. The physicians also performed an ultra-sound of her leg veins and found a large clot that extended up from her calf veins to her proximal veins.

In this case, a small clot likely formed in her calf veins during or soon after the surgical procedure. The clot then grew and extended into the veins above the knee. The clot did not completely block flow in the proximal vein and did not cause inflammation, therefore it did not cause any symptoms until two weeks after the operation when it broke off and traveled to the lung where the pulmonary embolism caused chest pain and breathing difficulties. Fortunately, the pulmonary embolism was recognized and responded to treatment, and Maya recovered. However, the pulmonary embolism could have been fatal.

Now consider the situation if the clot had totally blocked the vessel or caused the vessel to become inflamed.

> Maya, aged 69, had a gall bladder operation. She was recovering from the operation when, on the fourth day after surgery, she woke up with a painful, swollen, and discolored right leg. An ultrasound test was performed and showed that Maya had developed a thrombosis that extended from her calf veins into the vein behind her knee. She was treated and made a good recovery.
>
> In this case, Maya and her physicians were alerted to the presence of the clot much earlier because it produced severe leg symptoms.

Most leg vein clots start in the calf veins, and only a few grow into the proximal veins. In general, clots in calf veins do not produce serious complications, but they can be painful. However, if calf clots grow and extend into the deep veins above the knee (proximal veins), they can be dangerous because there is a risk that they can break off and cause serious pulmonary embolism. Similarly, the vast majority of superficial vein clots remain small and, although they can be painful, they are not life threatening. But again, a small percentage of superficial clots can grow and extend into the deep veins above the knee, although this extension is usually a slow process that can be detected easily and prevented before the clot passes into the deep veins. Superficial clots are usually very obvious to the patient because they cause a red, painful, cordlike line where the vein runs just under the skin. Unless they grow and extend into the deep veins, they do not break free and cause pulmonary emboli.

As we've already discussed, many venous clots cause no symptoms. Even large clots, if they do not obstruct the vein totally, might not cause symptoms. Even when a major vein is blocked, there are several smaller veins nearby that can begin to carry extra blood back to the heart to compensate for the blockage.

The common symptoms of deep venous clots, or deep vein thrombosis are:

- pain, tenderness, and/or swelling in the calf or thigh
- red or bluish discoloration of the calf or thigh
- chronic (long-term) leg swelling or discomfort

The clinical complications of venous clots can be divided into immediate and long term. The immediate complications are:

- acute pain that subsides within a few days with treatment
- symptoms of pulmonary or lung embolism

Pulmonary (Lung) Embolism

A lung embolus, or pulmonary embolism, is caused by a venous clot that breaks off and follows the path of the blood through the vein back to the right side of the heart, and from there, into the lung or pulmonary artery (see illustration on page 38). If the clot is very large, it can block blood flow into the lung arteries and cause severe breathing difficulties, or can even be fatal. Smaller lung emboli might cause chest pain, but many do not cause symptoms. With time, the emboli usually break up and disappear.

Almost all people who have pulmonary emboli also have evidence of clots in their legs when they are examined by special tests. However, only about one in three of these people have symptoms in their legs, meaning that those who seek medical care for symptoms of pulmonary embolism usually have had no symptoms from the clots in their legs.

Pulmonary Embolism

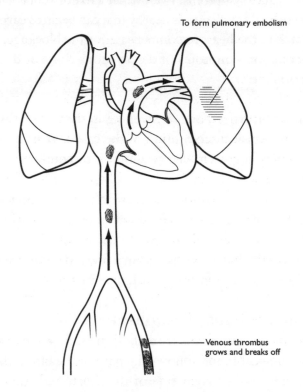

To form pulmonary embolism

Venous thrombus
grows and breaks off

Maya's story (page 35) is a typical example of pulmonary embolism and thrombosis without symptoms. You will recall that she developed sharp chest pain and difficulty in breathing two weeks after surgery. When she returned to hospital she was diagnosed with pulmonary embolism and, although she had no leg symptoms, a large clot was detected by ultrasonography (the test for venous thrombosis).

Although small emboli often don't produce any symptoms, larger ones usually do. The common symptoms of pulmonary embolism are:

- difficulty in breathing

- sharp chest pain that is aggravated by taking a deep breath
- blood that is coughed up from the lungs

If the pulmonary embolism is very large, it can cause light-headedness and fainting. In its most severe form, it can cause the heart to stop. In those circumstances, death usually occurs within the first twenty-four hours. Otherwise-healthy people can survive a very large pulmonary embolism, whereas people with heart or lung disease are much less likely to do so. Therefore, the most dangerous situations are those in which the pulmonary embolism is very large, blocking the main pulmonary artery, or if the person is already ill with heart or lung disease. Death occurs typically in one of two ways: either the clot is so large that it blocks all blood flow from the heart to the lungs, and cannot be dissolved quickly enough by any of the available blood-thinning or clot-dissolving treatments to prevent death, or a series of smaller emboli accumulate over the course of hours or days, with the same result.

The good news is that most people with pulmonary embolism do not die and respond well to treatment. Also, many pulmonary emboli, including potentially fatal emboli, can be anticipated because they occur in people with risk factors and *can therefore be prevented by using blood-thinning medication during the period of risk. Prevention, which is discussed in detail later, is the best course to take.* Death can be averted in most people if the embolism is diagnosed quickly and treated. Most often, lung embolism occurs in those who have just had surgery or who are ill and bedridden. In hospitals, measures are often taken to provide these patients with one of a variety of blood-thinning medications to prevent the occurrence of venous clots, and therefore reduce the likelihood of lung embolism.

Pulmonary embolism also can occur suddenly after people who have had a previous venous thrombosis stop taking blood thinners, and in those with blood abnormalities that predispose them to clotting. For this reason these "at risk" people are counseled about the symptoms of venous thrombosis and pulmonary embolism and are told to report to hospital if they develop suspicious symptoms. If this approach is followed, early diagnosis and prompt treatment can usually prevent death, even in people who develop large lung emboli. The diagnosis and treatment of pulmonary embolism is discussed later.

Long-Term Complications

With modern treatment, most people with venous clots recover completely or are left with mild swelling of the affected leg, and do not develop troublesome long-term complications. However, despite the best available treatment, some people do develop complications that can continue for their lifetime. These complications occur either because the initial clot damages venous valves, because it remains as a focus for further clotting, or because the risk factor that led to the first episode of clotting remains and leads to further clotting. The main long-term complications of venous clots are:

- persistent pain and swelling of the leg that can be permanent
- pulmonary hypertension
- further episodes of clotting in veins or in lung arteries

Persistent Leg Swelling and Discomfort (Post-Thrombotic Syndrome)

Betty, aged 54, worked as a supervisor in a clothing store. She was well and active, playing golf twice a week, when out of the blue she developed a deep vein thrombosis in her right leg. She had pain in the calf and thigh and marked swelling of her entire leg. An ultrasound examination of the leg showed a clot that had extended into the thigh vein and up into the groin area. She was treated with a blood thinner and the pain improved over the next three days, although the swelling improved only slightly. With further improvement in symptoms, Betty returned to limited activities. She began to walk around her house after a week and then ventured outside for short walks. The symptoms continued to improve although the swelling persisted and was more marked after she had been on her feet for more than an hour. She was advised to continue to take short walks and to be active.

After three months she had returned to near-normal activity. The acute pain in her leg was no longer present, but she had leg swelling that was much worse at the end of the day when she had been on her feet and that was accompanied by a heaviness and ache in her calf. She also noticed the appearance of prominent veins over her groin area and behind her knee. She was advised to elevate her leg when possible and was fitted with a compression stocking, which she was told to put on after her morning shower and to remove when she returned from work. At first, she wore the stocking intermittently, because it made her leg perspire, but after finding that it controlled her swelling and relieved the dull ache in her calf after a day at work, or a round of golf, she wore it during most of the day, taking it off when she returned home in the late afternoon.

After four months she realized the stocking was not helping her as much as previously and was informed that it needed replacing because it had lost its tension. After a year, she noticed that small networks of veins and brown spots had begun to appear on the inside of her ankle. She had gained some weight and noticed that she had lost some of her previous fitness when playing her usual game of golf. She went for dietary counseling and began an exercise program to strengthen her legs and improve cardiovascular fitness.

Two years later, Betty is living with her post-thrombotic syndrome. She wears a compression stocking during the day, has lost weight and regained her fitness, and works a full day and enjoys golf. Her right leg is more swollen than the left and she does have some aching after vigorous activity, but has learned that activity is good for her and does much more good than harm. She knows that her symptoms will persist for the rest of her life, but she has accepted this and lives a full life.

In some people, clots in the legs can damage the valves in the leg veins. The normal function of the valves in our leg prevents blood from pooling in the ankles when we stand up. When a person is lying down or horizontal, blood in the veins flows slowly toward the heart, and the venous valves are open because the pressure below the valve is slightly higher than the pressure above the valve. However, when we stand up, the valves close as soon as there is a pressure buildup above the valves. The closed veins prevent the blood from pooling in the leg veins. In this normal circumstance, when calf muscles contract, they squeeze blood up toward the heart. When the muscles relax, the valves close and prevent the blood from draining back toward the ankle.

However, when a venous clot occurs, it can become entangled in the delicate valves and distort them, thereby destroying their function. In this case, when the calf muscles contract, the blood begins to move upward in the direction of the heart, but then drains back toward the ankle when the contracting muscle relaxes. This process can be likened to a hose squirting water vertically—the water squirts up, but then it comes flowing down.

The result of this damage to the venous valves is chronic leg swelling and discomfort in the legs, called post-thrombotic syndrome. Not all venous clots result in this syndrome—the damage to the valve or valves has to be extensive in order to produce scarring of the valves to the point where they cannot function effectively. However, once it has developed, the process can become progressive. Destruction of the valves in one area by the clot can lead to an increase in the pressure on valves below those that have sustained the damage. The vein below the damaged valve can become distended or dilated, interfering with valve function to the point where the valves cannot close efficiently.

During the course of months and years, the increase in pressure in the veins around the ankle and lower leg (where the pressure increase is greatest) causes them to distend. Moreover, it causes the small microscopic vessels that drain into the veins to break and bleed—a process that produces tiny red spots that eventually merge and turn brown. The chronic increase in pressure in the veins forces fluid out of the vessels and leads to leg and ankle swelling that is typically worse at the end of the day (because the person has been upright) and is improved by the morning after a night's sleep. The buildup of fluid (known as *edema*) can cause a feeling of heaviness and even severe aching, which is most marked after long periods of standing or walking and relieved by lying down or elevating the affected leg.

In some very uncommon cases, post-thrombotic syndrome can be further complicated by the formation of ulcers that appear on the skin's surface. Typically, they occur above the inner ankle when the blood flow to the skin is most severely limited. The skin is often pigmented, or discolored, because of recurrent small bleeds from the thin-walled veins that are

Coping with post-thrombotic syndrome

Deep vein thrombosis can be complicated by lifelong leg swelling and discomfort; however, wearing properly fitted compression stockings can often control the symptoms. The stockings lose their elasticity after about four months and need to be replaced. It is important not to give in to the discomfort, but to live with and control it. People with post-thrombotic syndrome sometimes reduce their level of activity, gain weight, lose fitness, and become semi-invalids. The pain and discomfort after activity is temporary and does not cause permanent damage. Maintaining muscle strength and ideal body weight is important because a strong calf muscle is required to help pump the blood in the leg up to the heart and an increase in abdominal fat can impair the return of blood from the leg to the heart.

distended due to the increased venous pressure. Often the ulcer is precipitated by a mild injury to the area, from an ill-fitting boot for example. Usually, this type of ulceration can be avoided by the use of compression stockings and by avoiding injury to the leg.

Pulmonary Hypertension

An uncommon long-term complication of pulmonary or lung embolism is a condition called pulmonary hypertension, the buildup of blood pressure in the arteries of the lung due to a large clot. This condition is similar to the more common type of high blood pressure in the arterial circulation that your doctor measures when you get a checkup. However, the pressure buildup from pulmonary hypertension occurs in the pulmonary circulation, the arteries between the heart and the lung.

Fortunately, the development of pulmonary hypertension is fairly rare, occurring in about one in 100 cases of pulmonary embolism. The symptoms of pulmonary hypertension are:

- progressive shortness of breath, first during exertion and then at rest
- feeling lightheaded and, in severe cases, fainting

Pulmonary hypertension from large emboli that have not yet broken up (called thromboembolic pulmonary hypertension) used to be a fatal disorder but can now be treated surgically by removing the clots from the main lung arteries (see Chapter Six). The operation is quite specialized and is performed only in a limited number of medical centers. Most people make a good recovery.

Recurrent Clotting

The other long-term complication of venous clots is further episodes of clotting in the veins or in lung arteries. These compli cations can be minimized, but not completely avoided, providing the initial episode is treated properly. Further episodes of clotting occur either because the initial clot has not completely broken up and, therefore, acts as a focus for new clotting, or because the condition that led to the first clot is still present.

Blood thinners are very effective at preventing further clots, but since these drugs can cause bleeding and be inconvenient to use, many people opt to stop treatment after six months or more, and are then at risk of a second episode of clotting. Fortunately, new clots that occur can be readily treated. People who suffer a first episode of clotting often ask, "What can I do to prevent a second clot from forming?" "Is there something I should or shouldn't eat?" "Will exercise prevent recurrent clotting?"

The likelihood of developing a second clot during treatment with blood thinners is very low provided that the dosage of coumarin (the drug used to prevent clotting) is adequately controlled. However, as stated above, many people opt to stop anticoagulant treatment after months or years. In this circumstance, the risk of clotting is reduced by making sure that methods of prevention are used when the person is exposed to a high-risk situation, such as surgery or medical illness.

The recurrence can take the form of a second clot, in the same leg or the other leg, or it can take the form of a pulmonary embolism. The symptoms of recurrent clots and emboli are similar to those of a first episode of clotting. This issue of recurrent clots will be discussed when we consider the treatment and prevention of venous clots.

Venous Clots at Other Sites

While the most common site for venous clotting is in the legs, clots can form in veins in other parts of the body; for example in the veins of the arm, in the brain (cerebral veins), in the veins draining blood from the intestines (called mesenteric veins), and less commonly in other veins. Of these, clots in the arm veins occur most often, and those in the brain and intestines are potentially the most serious.

The mechanisms involved in the formation of all venous clots are similar, but the risk factors for these types of clots are different from those associated with clots in leg veins.

Arm Vein Clots

Clots in the veins of the arm occur most commonly in association with the presence of intravenous (IV) catheters that are kept in place to deliver treatments. For example, people being treated for cancer can have an IV in place for long periods in order to receive chemotherapy. This risk from the IV catheter is in addition to the underlying risk of venous clotting from the cancer itself.

Arm vein clots can also form in people who use their affected arm for repetitive activities, such as racquet sports. This type of arm vein thrombus is sometimes called "effort thrombosis." In others, there is no obvious cause and, in some of these cases, blood testing reveals an associated clotting defect in the person's blood.

The cause of thrombosis in those using intravenous catheters is irritation and damage to the inner lining of the arm vein produced by the catheter. In the case of effort thrombosis, the arm vein is injured as a result of it being pinched as it passes through a narrow opening between the muscles of the neck, collarbone, and first rib to enter the chest cavity.

When a clot occurs in an arm vein, it can cause swelling in the arm and pain or discomfort in the region of the upper arm or shoulder. The swelling can be quite severe and involve the hand as well as the forearm. The treatment is similar to that of leg vein thrombosis (See Chapter Six).

Although lung or pulmonary embolism can occur when emboli break off from an arm vein clot and travel to the lung, this complication occurs much less commonly than with clots in the veins of the leg.

Cerebral Vein Clots

Clots in the cerebral or brain veins are also rare, but they can be serious. In the past, they were seen with severe ear infections, but because of the availability of powerful antibiotics, ear infection is an uncommon cause. Now, cerebral vein clots are usually associated with pregnancy or occur just after the birth of a baby, or with the use of estrogen for contraception or hormone replacement therapy. Cerebral vein clots often occur in combination with the blood abnormalities that have already been discussed.

These cerebral vein clots can cause a type of stroke by blocking the outflow of blood from the affected area of the brain. Cerebral vein clots can also cause severe headache and blurring of vision. Blood wells up behind the clot and interferes with the normal circulation to the brain, and thereby damages the brain tissue. Fortunately, if treated early, the damage to the brain is usually not permanent. Cerebral vein clots are a much less common cause of stroke than clots in the arteries of the brain, which are the most common cause of stroke. The diagnosis of cerebral venous thrombosis is made using special imaging tests of the brain—computerized tomography (CT) scan or magnetic resonance imaging (MRI).

Without treatment, permanent damage to the brain was the rule for patients who developed clots in the cerebral veins. However, the blood-thinning medications now available, known as anticoagulants, are very effective. With appropriate treatment, most people recover completely from these types of clots. People who suffer one cerebral vein clot and recover are fearful of developing a second clot. Fortunately, the news for these people is good. Recurrent cerebral venous clotting is very unusual provided that precipitating factors are avoided. Estrogen should not be used and the possibility of future pregnancies should be considered only after discussion with a specialist—a hematologist, for example, or obstetrician specializing in the field.

Other Venous Clots
Even less commonly, clots can also occur in the veins of the intestines, eyes, kidneys, or liver. These clots are very unusual and potentially dangerous. They usually occur as a complication of some other disease.

- Clots in the intestines can occur in people with infections in their abdominal cavity and can cause abdominal pain and diarrhea.

- Clots in the back of the eye (retina) usually occur in people with high blood pressure and cause blurring of vision.
- Clots in the kidneys usually occur in people with other forms of kidney disease or those with cancer of the kidney. Unlike the other forms of unusual blood clots, those in the kidney veins can also break off to become a lung embolism.
- Liver clots usually occur in people with blood disorders. They cause abdominal pain, enlargement of the liver and spleen, and fluid accumulation in the abdomen.

Leg vein clots are by far the most common, accounting for more than 95 percent of all clots. Arm vein clots are much less common, whereas clots at the other sites are rare and make up only about 1 percent of all vein clots.

FOUR

Diagnosis of Venous Clots

The symptoms of deep venous thrombosis of the leg (leg pain and leg swelling) and of pulmonary embolism (chest pain and shortness of breath) can be caused by a variety of different conditions other than venous thrombosis or pulmonary embolism. For example, leg pain and swelling can be caused by an inflamed or injured muscle, a cyst behind the knee, knee joint problems, inflamed varicose veins, a torn tendon or muscle, cellulitis (an infection of fatty tissue just under the skin) of the leg, and a variety of other conditions. Chest pain and/or shortness of breath can be caused by a chest infection, bronchitis, a pneumothorax (ruptured air space of the lung, commonly called "collapsed" lung), heart disease, and many other lung disorders.

Up until about forty years ago, when faced with a person with possible venous thrombosis or pulmonary embolism, physicians were forced to rely on their clinical judgment and a number of unreliable tests. These diagnostic tests not only failed to correctly diagnose some people who had venous thrombosis or pulmonary embolism, but also misdiagnosed many. As a result, many patients who did not have venous or lung clots were unnecessarily treated with blood thinners. Initially, the diagnostic tests were complicated. In recent years they have been simplified so that a clinical diagnosis of venous thrombosis or pulmonary embolism can be easily confirmed or eliminated by using safe and reliable tests. These diagnostic tests are now always used to confirm whether people with suggestive symptoms do or do not have venous clots or lung emboli.

Diagnosing Deep Vein Thrombosis

The most useful test for diagnosing venous clots is compression ultrasonography, also called Venous Doppler and Color Doppler. This test is painless, available in most hospitals, and does not cause any complications. Some tests used to diagnose a variety of conditions carry small risks of their own, but this test does not. The test is performed by examining the veins in the leg using an ultrasound probe that transmits images of the vein onto a screen (like radar). The images are then interpreted by the ultrasound technician and confirmed by a specialist physician. When the probe is placed on the skin over the vein and artery, the images are transmitted as open vessels. When light pressure is applied, the normal vein collapses under the pressure. The artery remains open because it can withstand the light pressure. When the vein is filled with clot it does not collapse under light pressure and remains open.

If a clot is seen in a vein above the knee, a diagnosis of venous clot can be made with certainty because in these veins, the test is very reliable—which is important because it is clots in these proximal veins that are apt to cause the most problems. Treatment can then be started to prevent the clot from growing and breaking off to form emboli to the lungs. However, the ultrasound test might not always detect small clots in the veins below the knee (calf veins) Therefore, if a clot is not seen, a diagnosis of a clot in these calf veins cannot be ruled out with absolute certainty. The ultrasound test is less reliable in calf veins because these veins are much smaller than proximal veins, and the clots that form in calf veins can be very small. Small calf vein clots are not dangerous provided they do not grow and extend into the larger veins above the knee.

If the ultrasound test shows no clots in these veins below the knee, the strategy is to then follow up with an additional compression ultrasonography test in five to seven days. This approach works because:

- Clots not seen on ultrasound are not clinically important; that is they do not cause real problems—most importantly, pulmonary embolism—unless they continue to grow and extend into the veins above the knee, and
- Providing these clots have not extended into the veins above the knee within seven days of the original checkup, then they are very unlikely to do so.

For this reason, if the ultrasound test initially has a negative result, it is an accepted and safe practice to re-examine the person with the clot again in seven days. If no clot is visible at that point, then we can be confident that a dangerous venous clot did not cause the leg pain. If the original negative test becomes positive at the re-examination, then we conclude that the original symptoms were in fact due to a calf vein clot that has now extended into the vein above the knee, and appropriate treatment is then given to prevent further extension.

The need to perform a follow-up venous Doppler (if the initial one is normal) can be inconvenient—although it is safe. Recently, two new approaches have been introduced that overcome the need for a repeat test in many patients. These approaches are:

- Performing a careful clinical evaluation that allows people with suspected venous thrombosis to be classified as having low or intermediate probability for venous clots.

If the venous ultrasound is normal, further testing is not required providing the person is rated as having low probability for thrombosis.

- Performing a D-dimer test, which is a blood test. If the D-dimer test is negative in a person with a normal venous ultrasound, the diagnosis of venous thrombosis can be excluded without the need for further testing.

The D-dimer test measures tiny particles of fibrin (a component of the blood clot) that are present in people who have clots and other illnesses. A negative D-dimer means that clotting has not occurred. Therefore, if a person shows no signs of leg clots on the compression ultrasound test and also has a negative D-dimer test, this is proof that no clot is present, and a follow-up examination is not necessary. However, the D-dimer test cannot be used by itself to establish a diagnosis because many other medical problems can cause a positive result, including such things as infection. Therefore, when the D-dimer test shows a positive result, we always have to perform further testing.

Occasionally, the ultrasound might be difficult to interpret or is negative in a person who has classical symptoms of a venous clot, making the physician highly suspicious that a clot is in fact present. If either of these two circumstances occur, it might be necessary to perform an X-ray of the legs after injecting a dye that outlines the veins. Dye—containing a material that is opaque to X-rays—is injected into a vein in the foot a few minutes before the X-ray is taken. The dye mixes with the blood in the veins, which are outlined and seen on the X-ray. This test is called a venogram and can usually resolve any diagnostic uncertainty in these problematic cases.

Although a venogram is straightforward and definitive, allowing the veins and any clots to be seen clearly, it is not performed in all cases because it can be painful and is risky for people who have kidney disease. Instead, the test is limited to those cases that cannot be diagnosed using the painless and easier tests.

Carol, a 26-year-old woman, developed pain in her left calf that gradually became more severe. It was associated with swelling in her left leg from the ankle to just below the knee. She went to the emergency department of a nearby hospital where she told the physician examining her that she had been on an oral contraceptive for one year. He examined her leg and noted that there was tenderness in the back of her calf and that the left leg had a dusky bluish tinge. An ultrasound was performed and this showed a large clot extending up into her thigh vein. She was started on blood thinners, and her symptoms gradually improved over a week.

The clinical probability of venous clotting was high because the symptoms were classical. Although Carol's symptoms were confined to her calf, the clot involved her proximal veins and extended up to the groin—a common scenario in which the site of the symptoms does not reflect the extent of the clot.

Let's now modify Carol's story and her ultrasound results to make an important point.

Margaret, a 37-year-old woman, developed pain in her left calf. It was associated with *mild* swelling of her left ankle. (Note, Margaret's symptoms were as severe as Carol's.) She went to the emergency department of a nearby hospital where the physician examined her leg and noted that there was slight tenderness in the back of her calf. The result of her ultrasound was normal. The physician thought that a calf vein thrombus was likely because there was no other explanation for the symptoms, and

Margaret was on the pill. He performed a D-dimer test that was positive. (Remember, a D-dimer test is useful when it is negative, because such a result excludes thrombosis. A positive test is less useful because it cannot be used to make a diagnosis of leg vein thrombosis.) Five days later, her physician repeated the venous ultrasound test and it was still normal. By that time Margaret's symptoms had subsided and she was given a clean slate of health.

The normal, repeat venous ultrasound did not exclude the presence of a small calf vein thrombosis, but it did exclude a dangerous thrombus or one that might become dangerous by growing into the proximal veins. The physician might have considered performing a venogram if Margaret's symptoms had progressed, because if her symptoms had been caused by a calf vein thrombus, they would respond to blood thinners.

Diagnosis of Pulmonary (Lung) Embolism

As is the case with venous clots, all of the symptoms caused by pulmonary or lung embolism can be caused by other disorders including pneumonia, viral pleurisy, bronchitis, pneumothorax, pulled chest wall muscle, heart attack, or anxiety. Therefore, the clinical suspicion of lung embolism must also be confirmed using one of a variety of diagnostic tests.

In general, these tests are more complicated than those used to diagnose venous clots. Four tests are most commonly used. Which tests are used in any given situation is a decision that depends on the preferences of your physician and the availability of the tests themselves. The tests are:

Ventilation and Perfusion (V/Q) Scan

There are two components of this test. A ventilation (V) scan and a perfusion (Q) scan. By performing both types of scans, the airflow in the lungs is compared to the blood flow. If pulmonary embolism is present, blood flow is reduced and air flow is normal. This is in contrast with most other lung conditions, where the airflow is reduced and blood flow is affected less.

The V/Q scan is available in most hospitals. The tests are similar to a chest X-ray in that images of the lung are snapped by a camera and are recorded on photographic film (like X-ray film).

- First, the ventilation (V) scan, which measures the flow of air into the air spaces of the lung, is performed. To accomplish this, the person taking the test breathes a radioactive gas from a tube. This gas, which is harmless and leaves the body quickly, enters the air spaces of the lungs. Its distribution in the lung is captured by the camera and recorded on X-ray film. If there are sections of the lungs that are not filled with gas, the image seen on the X-ray film shows gaps.
- Then, the perfusion scan that measures blood flow in the pulmonary arteries. Radioactive particles are injected into the bloodstream. These particles, which are also harmless and rapidly dissolved by the body, outline the distribution of blood flow to the pulmonary arteries. The image is captured on the camera and recorded on X-ray film.

The ventilation and perfusion scans are then compared to see if there is a difference between the areas of airflow and those of blood flow.

The test is very useful if it is either normal, indicating no blood clot, or very abnormal, indicating a definite blood clot. However, V/Q scans can sometimes be hard to interpret (even for doctors!) because many types of lung disease, if present, can alter the findings. When such uncertainty occurs, other tests are performed to determine the diagnosis. Because of this, the V/Q scan is being gradually replaced by newer tests.

Spiral Computed Tomography (CT) Scan

Spiral computed tomography (also known as a helical CT scan) is a relatively new alternative test used by many doctors to investigate pulmonary embolism. During this test, an X-ray tube rotates continuously around a patient as the patient is smoothly moved in the CT scanner through the X-ray scan field. This produces a corkscrew or helical-like path. The CT images are usually taken during a single breath-hold. Pulmonary emboli are detected as filling spaces in the lung arteries. Spiral CT scanning is now replacing the V/Q scan in many hospitals because, when it is positive, the spiral CT confirms a diagnosis of lung embolism.

Pulmonary Angiogram

Like the venogram, the lung angiogram is the most reliable test to identify clots in the arteries of the lungs. A negative result from a pulmonary angiogram excludes the diagnosis of pulmonary embolism—however, the test is invasive and is used only if less invasive tests are inconclusive.

The test involves passing a catheter through a large vein in the groin into the right side of the heart, and injecting dye into the catheter. The dye outlines the pulmonary arteries, and the image is recorded by an X-ray. Because the test is somewhat painful and carries a small risk, it is performed only in unusual cases and when other tests yield uncertain results.

D-dimer

As with venous clots, the D-dimer blood test, when it is negative, can help to exclude a diagnosis of lung embolism.

Finally, because pulmonary emboli are often the result of pieces of clot that have broken off from larger clots in the legs, a compression ultrasound of the legs that proves positive for leg clots can support a diagnosis of pulmonary embolism. A negative ultrasound test, however, does not exclude a diagnosis of lung embolism. This is because the venous clot from which the embolism originated might have broken up and therefore might not be present when the person develops symptoms of lung embolism. In addition, about 10 percent of pulmonary emboli are thought to arise from veins in other parts of the body.

Taras, a 55-year-old man who had recently undergone a successful hernia repair, developed sudden sharp chest pain and difficulty breathing. He was re-admitted to hospital, and a V/Q scan showed a picture that was classical for pulmonary embolism. The diagnosis was made, and he was treated successfully with blood thinners.

This was an easy case to diagnose. However, most cases are not so easy. If Taras had vague symptoms of chest pain and the V/Q scan was not diagnostic, then other tests would be required. A negative D-dimer test would make a diagnosis of pulmonary embolism very unlikely. On the other hand, if the D-dimer test was positive, Taras would have been referred to a hospital that performs spiral CT scans.

Making a diagnosis of pulmonary embolism is easy when the test results are clear and either positive or negative. However, in many cases, the initial V/Q test results are not clear and other tests have to be performed to either make or exclude a diagnosis of pulmonary embolism. The introduction of the spiral CT scan and D-dimer has simplified diagnosis.

FIVE

Prevention of Clots in Veins and Lung Arteries

The most effective way to prevent death and disability from leg clots and lung emboli is to prevent the clots themselves. The decision to use preventative methods and the choice of which methods to use is made by your physician or surgeon, so this chapter will be brief and limited to the principles of prevention.

Prevention, also known as prophylaxis, should be used in all hospitalized patients who are considered moderate or high risk for developing venous thrombosis. The use of prophylaxis in such patients reduces the risk of developing venous clots and lung emboli by about 70 percent. It also reduces death from lung emboli by 70 percent. Although many patients develop venous clots and lung emboli outside of the hospital setting, most deaths from pulmonary embolism occur in hospitalized patients. The majority of these deaths can be avoided, thanks to a number of highly effective and safe methods of prevention.

Prevention of Venous Clots in Hospitalized Patients

There are now several very effective methods for preventing clots in veins and lung arteries and their use is strongly encouraged in patients with risk factors. Prevention of venous clots should be considered in all hospitalized patients who are high risk for thrombosis. The high risk conditions were discussed in detail in Chapter Two. They include:

- major surgery, especially hip and knee surgery, cancer surgery and any other surgery that requires prolonged post-operative bed rest
- major trauma to chest, legs, and pelvis (although any serious trauma is a risk factor)
- prolonged immobility due to any illness or surgery
- major medical illness requiring hospitalization, especially due to heart disease and severe lung disease
- previous venous thrombosis

As a general rule, all patients who have surgery under general anesthesia which lasts for half an hour or longer and who require bed rest after surgery are considered at risk and should receive prophylaxis. The risk of developing venous clots increases with the length and extensiveness of surgery. For example, a minor operation to remove a cyst on the arm would be considered low risk, but an operation to remove a tumor in the abdomen is considered high risk.

Since the risk of thrombosis is usually transient and limited to the post-operative period, the duration of prevention is short (days or weeks). In general prophylaxis should be continued until the patient has returned to near normal activity. Two types of approaches are used to prevent blood clots: blood thinners (anticoagulants) that are used in low doses to slow the clotting process, and physical methods to prevent pooling of blood in leg veins.

Blood Thinners and Movement

In most cases, blood thinners are used to prevent clots in patients at risk because they are more reliable and convenient to use than the most effective physical methods. Although blood thinners can produce some bleeding in a patient having surgery, the risk is reduced markedly by lowering the dose and by avoiding use during surgery itself. There is now no question that, in most cases, the benefits of prevention with blood thinners outweigh the small risk of bleeding when given to sick medical patients and high and moderate risk surgical patients.

With certain high risk procedures (extensive plastic surgery, major internal trauma, spinal surgery), the risk of bleeding even with low doses of blood thinners is too high to warrant their use. In those patients, prevention focuses on physical approaches that prevent the pooling of blood in the legs. There are two ways of preventing pooling in leg veins. The first and simplest is to use elasticized stockings; the second is to use mechanical compression of the calf. Simple elasticized stockings are not as effective as blood thinners or as the mechanical devices. Pooling of blood in leg veins is also prevented by early mobilization and this is encouraged in all patients.

Although preventive measures should be used in moderate and high-risk patients, because their benefits clearly outweigh their risks, their use is not required in low-risk situations. In general, low-risk patients are those who have only minor surgery which lasts less than 30 minutes. They are able to walk without difficulty soon after surgery and should be encouraged to do so.

As already discussed, in most cases, low doses of a blood thinner are used. In surgical patients or those who experience major trauma, the blood thinner is usually started when the risk of bleeding has abated. The risk of serious bleeding usually subsides six or more hours after surgery, but may not abate for a day or more after severe trauma. The risk of bleeding is very low in the absence of surgery or trauma, so blood thinners can be started without delay in individuals who are immobilized for reasons other than surgery or trauma. Blood thinners are continued for at least the length of the hospital stay. For patients who remain at risk after leaving the hospital, the blood thinner is continued until the patients are no longer at risk. For some patients, the period of increased risk can be as long as 30 days, but, for most, it is 5 to 10 days. In certain circumstances, a blood thinner might be used before surgery, in very low doses.

There are four blood thinners available for use for the prevention or treatment of venous thrombosis. These are heparin, low-molecular-weight heparin, fondaparinux, and warfarin. Other new blood thinners are being developed. Details on these anticoagulants are discussed in Chapter 6.

Anticoagulants Used to Prevent Clots

Anticoagulant (Blood Thinner)	Method of administration
low doses of heparin	injection twice or three times daily
low-molecular-weight heparin	injection once daily
fondaparinux	injection once daily
warfarin	orally (by mouth) once daily

The mechanical device that is used to prevent pooling of blood in leg veins is an inflatable cuff that squeezes the muscles of the calf, or calf and thigh, periodically. By so doing, it pumps blood out of the leg and prevents pooling. The device is removed when the patient gets out of bed and should be replaced as soon as the patient returns to bed. This is not always possible in a busy hospital setting and therefore in most cases blood thinners are preferred. The mechanical device can be placed over an elastic stocking that can continue to be worn when the patient gets out of bed.

Prevention of Venous Clots Outside the Hospital Setting

People with Previous Venous Clots

People who have had an episode of unprovoked thrombosis are at increased risk of a second clot when they discontinue warfarin. This risk can be reduced if they receive prophylaxis with blood thinners whenever exposed to a high or even moderate risk situation. These situations might include: a leg injury that requires the use of a splint; the necessity for a long-distance flight; the contracting of a chest infection of other medical illness that requires bed rest.

Long-distance Travel

Airline thrombosis has received a lot of publicity recently and, understandably, some people who are about to go on long trips become concerned about developing venous clots. Long-distance air travel is a very minor risk factor, unless the traveler has other risk factors, such as prior venous clots, a major medical illness, severe varicose veins, or a familial blood disorder that predisposes him or her to thrombosis. Short trips don't appear to increase the risk of venous clots, but trips over six hours do increase the risk.

Long-distance travelers are encouraged to move around the cabin, flex their leg muscles, and drink plenty of non-alcoholic beverages. Flexing of calf and thigh muscles can be performed without the need to get out of your seat. If more protection is required, simple elasticized calf-length stocking can be used. These have been shown to be effective. In one clinical trial aspirin was not effective. The use of an injectable anticoagulant is very effective for preventing airline thrombosis, but this approach is limited to the very high risk person. In very high risk travelers— a person with a history of unprovoked venous thrombosis, for example—a blood thinner such as low-molecular-weight heparin or fondaparinux would be prescribed. This would be injected just under the skin before leaving for the airport on both the outgoing and return trip. If high risk people are already being treated with warfarin, and their level of anticoagulation (blood thinning) is appropriate, they are well protected and do not need additional measures.

Healthy women who are taking estrogens for contraception or hormone replacement do not need to stop estrogens or take extra precautions when they fly. Their risk of developing blood clots is extremely low, provided that they don't have other risk factors. If they are concerned about developing clots they should exercise their legs and maintain good hydration. Similarly, pregnant women with an uncomplicated pregnancy are low risk for developing venous clots during long flights. If they have significant leg swelling, they should consider wearing elasticized stockings. If, however, a pregnant woman has inherited thrombophilia, or a woman on hormone replacement therapy has severe varicose veins or is immobile because of a chronic illness, she should see her physician. More active measures might need to be taken—either elastic stockings or, in the very high-risk person, an injection with a blood thinner.

S I X

Treatment

O nce the diagnosis of venous clots or pulmonary embolism has been made, there are a variety of treatments that will help prevent the clots from growing, assist the body to dissolve the clots, and stop clots from forming again. These treatments are highly effective; in other words, the vast majority of people with vein clots survive and most are left with no or only minimal disability.

Treatment can be divided into two stages: immediate treatment of venous clots and lung emboli, and continuing treatment of these clots. Once treatment with blood thinners (known as anticoagulants) or fibrinolytic or clot-dissolving drugs (clot busters) is started, the chances of survival are excellent. Therefore, it is important to recognize the symptoms of venous clots or lung emboli so that the diagnosis can be confirmed and treatment started without delay.

The objective of *immediate* treatment is to:

- prevent the growth of the vein clots
- prevent clots from breaking off and becoming pulmonary emboli
- prevent death from lung emboli
- help the body dissolve any lung emboli that might be present
- relieve the symptoms caused by both conditions

The objective of *continuing* treatment is to:

- prevent repeat venous clots and lung emboli
- relieve the symptoms caused by post-thrombotic syndrome

As discussed in Chapter Three, post-thrombotic syndrome is a condition that causes chronic pain and swelling of the affected leg. The symptoms arise from the destruction of the venous valves or the continuing obstruction of venous blood flow in the leg by a previous clot. Typically, different drugs are used for immediate and for long-term treatment.

Immediate treatment of an acute episode of leg vein thrombosis or pulmonary embolism is either with an injectable blood thinner, or with the so-called clot-buster medications that act directly to break up a clot. These powerful medications are given by injection and act immediately.

For continuing treatment, which usually takes place outside the hospital, prescribed anticoagulant medications are taken orally or—less frequently—are self-injected, similar to the self-injection of insulin by people with diabetes.

First, let's discuss the blood-thinning medications.

Blood Thinners

The medical name for blood thinners is anticoagulants. These agents do not actually "thin" the blood, but rather slow blood clotting and so prevent clots from growing or reforming. Four different kinds of blood thinners are in current use for the treatment and prevention of venous thrombosis:

- heparin
- low-molecular-weight heparin
- fondaparinux (a recent addition)
- warfarin, also known as Coumadin

Heparin is given by intravenous injection (into a vein), low-molecular-weight heparin (LMWH) and fondaparinux are given by subcutaneous injection (by needle under the skin), and warfarin is taken by mouth. Since blood thinners slow blood clotting, it is not surprising that their most common (although still rare) complication is bleeding. The bleeding is not usually serious and consists of nosebleeds, bruising, or bleeding gums after brushing the teeth. However, serious bleeding can occur after an operation if blood thinners are used in high doses within a few days of surgery and if the patient suffers from an internal disorder that is prone to bleed, such as an ulcer, or from a kidney stone or cancer. As noted in Chapter Five, blood thinners are used in low doses to prevent venous clots after surgery. When used in low doses, the risk of bleeding is minimal.

The correct way of prescribing blood thinners is to determine a dose that slows clotting enough to prevent thrombosis, but not so much so that they cause bleeding. Fortunately, if given in the correct way, bleeding is not common with these drugs. Doctors have lots of experience with heparin, LMWH, and warfarin. A new drug, fondaparinux, has been introduced only recently. Because acetylsalicylic acid (aspirin or ASA) is not an anticoagulant and is much less effective for the prevention and treatment of venous clots and lung emboli, it is not recommend in place of anticoagulants.

Other new blood thinners are now being developed. The two oldest are heparin and warfarin, both of which have been a staple of treatment for more than fifty years.

Heparin

When used to treat people with blood clots, heparin is given by an infusion into the vein, known as intravenous infusion. As a result, its use is mostly confined to those people who are in the hospital. Heparin is given also by subcutaneous injection when

Is heparin safe?

Although heparin is derived from animal tissues, there is no need for concern about the safety of this treatment. After decades of use in many millions of people, there is no evidence that heparin or its derivative, LMWH, have been responsible for transmitting any animal diseases to people.

used to prevent thrombosis in people with high-risk conditions. Heparin is a natural product: it is a long-chained negatively charged sugar.

Heparin was discovered by a medical student (Jay McLean at John's Hopkins University) more than ninety years ago. McLean was experimenting with extracts of homogenized dog liver in the hope of finding a substance that *caused* clotting. Instead, he found a substance that *prevented* clotting and, since it was derived from the liver, it was named heparin (*hepar* is the Latin word for liver). Subsequently, commercial heparin has been extracted from pig gut by a process that has changed little in the last fifty years. First used in humans around 1940 by physicians in Canada and Sweden, heparin has proven invaluable to our health and has saved millions of lives. For example, without heparin, open-heart surgery or kidney dialysis could not have been developed and perfected.

Side Effects

Heparin is a so-called indirect blood thinner because it slows clotting by activating a natural anticlotting protein known as antithrombin that turns off the clotting mechanism. The main drawback of heparin is that the blood-thinning effect of a fixed dose is both unpredictable and differs from person to person. Consequently, this effect must be monitored, at least daily, by a blood test, known as the activated partial thromboplastin time (APTT). The dose is altered according to the result of the

APTT. This requirement for frequent blood test monitoring is tedious and restricts the use of heparin to an in-hospital setting.

The most common side effect of heparin and any of the anticoagulant medications is excessive bleeding. Because the action of these drugs is to reduce the blood's tendency to clot, this action can cause some excessive bleeding from time to time. Bleeding occurs most commonly if the person receiving the blood thinner has a source for bleeding; for example, has recently had surgery or trauma due to an accident, or if she or he has a kidney stone or stomach ulcer. Under these circumstances, bleeding can occur even if heparin and other blood thinners are given correctly. Bleeding can also occur without a provoking cause (such as surgery) if excessively high doses of the blood thinner are given—which is why it is important that the dosage of blood thinners be carefully controlled.

In general, this bleeding is little more than a nuisance, troublesome but not serious. For example, you may notice that you have an increased tendency to bruise, nosebleeds, bleeding gums when brushing your teeth, and bleeding at the site of injection. Normally, this type of bleeding does not require discontinuation of the treatment. More serious bleeding (which happens in about one in fifty people) most commonly occurs at the site of a wound or lesion, such as an ulcer, cancer, or kidney stone, and originates from the bowel, kidneys, or other internal organs. The most serious form of bleeding is into the brain, a complication that is usually restricted to elderly people, particularly those with high blood pressure or a previous history of stroke.

Ironically, heparin can sometimes cause thrombosis if its use is complicated by a condition known as heparin-induced thrombocytopenia (known as HIT), which is caused by antibodies that the body produces in response to heparin. Thrombosis can occur when heparin-dependent antibodies activate blood platelets that in turn set off an intense clotting process. Fortunately, thrombosis due to HIT is uncommon, occurring in about 1 in 100 people. If HIT occurs, heparin is stopped immediately and replaced by other more recently developed blood thinners.

Another complication of heparin is bone thinning (osteoporosis). This is a very rare complication and occurs only in about 2 in 100 people who are treated with heparin for at least two to three months. Fortunately, these drawbacks of heparin are much less with the new heparins, known as low-molecular-weight heparin (LMWH) and with the new, synthetic heparin-like product, fondaparinux.

Low-Molecular-Weight Heparin (LMWH)

Low-molecular-weight heparin is produced from heparin through a chemical process that reduces the size of the heparin molecule; molecules of LMWH are about one-third the size of the original heparin.

LMWH was discovered by chance in the 1970s and, after years of basic and clinical research, was introduced for treatment of humans in the 1990s. There are now a number of LMWH preparations licensed for use. These include enoxaparin, dalteparin, and tinzaparin. These preparations have several clear advantages over their predecessor.

First, the blood-thinning effect of low-molecular-weight heparin is more predictable, so regular blood testing—to measure the degree of thinning of the blood caused by the drug—is not required. To appreciate why the blood-thinning effect of LMWH is more predictable than that of heparin, it is important to understand that the reason for heparin's unpredictable effect is because its molecules are highly charged and therefore stick to various proteins in the bloodstream. The concentration (amount) of these proteins in the bloodstream increases to an unpredictable degree in people who are ill. As a result, the amount of heparin that is available to produce its blood-thinning effect is reduced to a variable degree in people with various illnesses (including thrombosis). LMWH is more predicable because, being smaller than heparin, the LMWH molecules are less sticky than heparin; therefore, most of the material injected is available to produce a blood-thinning effect. We'll talk more about the need for regular blood testing later in this chapter.

Second, LMWH is less likely than heparin to produce HIT. As already discussed, whereas thrombosis caused by HIT occurs in about 1 in 100 people treated with heparin for at least five days, it occurs only in about 1 in 500 people treated with LMWH. In this case, the reason for the lower risk is related to the fact that the smaller LMWH molecules do not stick as firmly to a protein that promotes the development of HIT antibodies.

Third, LMWH is about ten times less likely than heparin to produce bone thinning (osteoporosis). The reason is that LMWH sticks less strongly than heparin to the bone cells that trigger bone thinning. Actually, it is now known that when heparin sticks to bone cells, it stimulates the cells to release chemicals that both slow down bone formation and speed up bone loss.

Like heparin, LMWH must be given by injection under the skin (subcutaneous injection), but while heparin—if given subcutaneously—must be given twice daily, only one daily dose of LMWH is required. Finally, there is evidence that low-molecular-weight heparins are slightly more effective than heparin.

Side Effects

While LMWH is usually well tolerated by those who take them for either short- or long-term treatment, there are several potential side effects. There is, for example, a small risk of osteoporosis, or bone thinning, when LMWH is taken for several months, but this is much less common than is seen with heparin.

If you are taking these drugs for three months or longer, your doctor might ask you to have a bone density scan—a simple and painless procedure that will give plenty of warning if your bones are thinning in response to the medication. If the bone scan shows evidence of bone thinning, the drug can be stopped. Fortunately, once LMWH is stopped, not only is the process of bone thinning arrested, the condition of your bones gradually returns to the pre-treatment level.

There is still a small risk of heparin-induced thrombocytopenia with LMWH, but it is less likely than with heparin. For example, after at least five days of treatment with LMWH, the risk of HIT is between 1 in 100 and 1 in 1,000 depending on the disease being treated.

There are three low-molecular-weight heparins approved for use in North America: enoxaparin, dalteparin, and tinzaparin. More LMWH preparations are approved for use in Europe. Although produced by different processes, these various drugs are about the same size from a molecular standpoint, and there are no important differences between the LMWHs either in their beneficial or adverse effects.

Despite heparin's limitations in comparison to low-molecular-weight heparins, there are still some situations where your doctor might consider heparin to be the preferable treatment. For example, heparin is still the blood thinner of choice for safe cardiac bypass surgery, and might be preferred to LMWH for people with a very large lung embolism or for those who have kidney disease.

Fondaparinux

The newest blood thinner to become available is called fondaparinux. About twenty-five years ago, scientists discovered that the blood-thinning effect of both heparin and LMWH is produced by a small segment of these molecules. This segment is a five-sugar unit known as a pentasaccharide (penta = five, saccharide = sugar). After scientists worked out the chemical structure of this special blood-thinning segment, they set out to manufacture it. It took about twenty years of painstaking work but eventually fondaparinux was produced. The cost of production and clinical development was enormous—hundreds of millions of dollars. Fondaparinux is now approved in Canada and the U.S. for the prevention of blood clots after major orthopedic surgery and for the treatment of blood clots.

While fondaparinux produces its blood-thinning effects by a similar mechanism as LMWH and heparin, unlike both heparin and LMW heparin, fondaparinux is a synthetic compound. It is not derived from animal tissues. Since it is a small molecule, it does not bind to positively charged proteins in the blood, and therefore has a very predictable blood-thinning effect. It is given once daily by subcutaneous injection and, although like all blood thinners it can cause bleeding, it does not cause HIT (the most common non-bleeding side effect of heparin).

Studies have shown that fondaparinux is at least as effective as LMWH or heparin at preventing clotting for people at high risk of blood clots and for the treatment of blood clots. At present, experience with fondaparinux is more limited than heparin or LMWH, but its approval for clinical use provides doctors with yet another effective and safe alternative to prevent and treat blood clots.

Warfarin
Although there are three classes of blood thinners given by injection (heparin, LMWH, and fondaparinux), only one class of blood thinners is taken by mouth (oral anticoagulant). There

The discovery of coumarin

More than eighty years ago, coumarins were discovered by a Wisconsin scientist who isolated the compound from spoiled clover. The story goes that a farmer suspected the connection between feeding his cattle with spoiled sweet clover and their bleeding disorder. He traveled the many miles to Wisconsin in the depths of winter with a bag of the spoiled clover and a bucket of an affected cow's blood. It was a vacation day but, fortunately, the scientist was at work and so the coumarins were discovered.

Coumarins have been used as a rat poison for decades. Rudimentary clinical trials were performed with warfarin in the early 1940s. Subsequently, larger well-designed trials established warfarin and similar compounds (coumarins) as effective blood thinners, and they have been the mainstay of out-of-hospital treatment for more than sixty years. Now, millions of people are taking warfarin.

is an important need to develop new oral anticoagulants (see Disadvantages, below) and a number of large pharmaceutical companies are in the race. The one class of oral blood thinners currently available is called vitamin K antagonists (also known as coumarins), the most common of which is warfarin (commonly known by the trade name coumadin).

Because tablets are convenient, warfarin is the usual choice for continuing treatment to prevent further clotting—once patients have already received treatment for their immediate clotting problem.

Disadvantages

Despite its value, warfarin has significant disadvantages: it requires very careful blood monitoring and can be difficult to use in some people. Based on these difficulties and the widespread need for an oral blood thinner and the enormous improvement in drug development technology, its pre-eminent position as the only oral blood thinner is now being challenged by a number of new synthetic oral blood thinners, which are much easier to use. None of these new drugs is yet available for clinical use.

Warfarin is used for the treatment of blood clots in veins and for the prevention of stroke in patients with certain heart disorders. Some doctors also use warfarin to prevent vein clots after major orthopedic surgery. The main drawback to warfarin is the need for people taking it to have frequent blood tests (with the INR [International Normalized Ratio]—a method of measuring the thinness of blood that is used to determine the most appropriate dose of coumadin) and careful dose adjustment. Warfarin has a narrow therapeutic index—meaning that if under dosed, it loses effectiveness and if overdosed it leads to bleeding. The blood-thinning effect of warfarin is affected by changes in the vitamin K content of the diet, since warfarin produces this effect by counteracting vitamin K. Many drugs can also either increase or decrease the blood-thinning effect of warfarin. It takes about five days for warfarin to produce its required blood-thinning effect. Therefore, when used to treat people with blood clots, an injectable blood thinner and warfarin are started at the same time and when the blood-thinning warfarin effect is appropriate (usually five to six days), the injectable blood thinner is stopped. Warfarin is then continued for months to years.

Side effects of blood thinners

Medication	Bleeding	Heparin-induced thrombocytopenia	Osteoporosis (bone thinning)
heparin	yes	yes (3%)	yes, but uncommon, occurring only when treatment is continued for months
LMWH	yes	yes (less than 1%)	yes, but even less common than with heparin
fondaparinux	yes	not expected	not expected
warfarin (coumarins)	yes	no	no

One of the disadvantages of coumadin has been the need for people taking it to come into an office or hospital to have blood taken for INR testing. This inconvenience has been overcome by the introduction of a self-testing device similar to the glucometer used by diabetic patients. The device pricks the finger, then adds the drop of blood to a small cartridge that contains the reagents to measure the INR. The result is obtained within a minute. Although the device and the cartridge are more expensive than the standard test, many people consider the time saved and the empowerment provided worth the expense.

Clot Busters (Fibrinolytic Drugs)

Finally, another class of drugs used in the treatment of venous clots is the so-called "clot-busting" medications. As the name implies, the purpose of these medications is to attack and break up a clot that already exists. The medical term for clot-buster drugs is fibrinolytic agents. Clot busters include drugs such as tissue-plasminogen activator (tPA), tenectaplase, reteplase, and streptokinase.

Clot busters are more powerful than blood thinners. Whereas blood thinners slow clotting and prevent a clot from growing, clot busters actively and rapidly dissolve the clot. Therefore, they are much more powerful than blood-thinning medications. However, clot busters have a downside: they cause more bleeding than blood thinners. Because of this potential for bleeding, they are usually reserved for the largest and most life threatening of lung emboli. These are the same medications that people receive when they have a heart attack or, in some cases, a stroke—both caused by life-threatening clots that form in the arterial system. However, since more than 95 percent of patients with venous clots or lung emboli survive if blood thinners are used, the risk of causing excessive bleeding outweighs any small benefits in all but those people with very large lung emboli.

Drugs for immediate and continuing treatment of venous clots and lung emboli

Medication	Taken	Other names	Blood testing required	Out-of-hospital use	Comments
clot busters	intravenous infusion	fibrinolytic or thrombolytic agents	–	no	because of the risk of bleeding, clot busters are given only in the case of life-threatening lung emboli
heparin	intravenous infusion	Blood thinner or anticoagulant	yes	no	has largely been replaced by LMW heparin
LMWH	injection under the skin (subcutaneous injection)	Blood thinner or anticoagulant	no	yes	preferred over heparin because it can be given by subcutaneous injection without laboratory testing
Fondaparinux	injection under the skin (subcutaneous injection)	Blood thinner or anticoagulant	no	yes	has just been introduced. Has similar or perhaps improved benefit as LMW heparin
warfarin (coumarins)	by mouth (orally)	Blood thinner or anticoagulant	yes	yes	dose is adjusted by regular measurements with blood test (INR). Dosage control can be difficult. Home monitoring devices are now available.

Treatment of Venous Clots or Lung Emboli

When venous clots or lung emboli occur, it is important to start treatment promptly in order to prevent further complications. Treatment of clots of different types and locations occurs in two stages, from the first stage of initial symptoms to ongoing treatment that is usually required outside the hospital.

Deep Venous (Leg) Clots

After his morning walk, Bob, a 45-year-old stockbroker, noticed that his left leg was swollen. He thought little of it and went to work. The swelling became more marked, and he developed pain in the calf and behind his left knee. He saw his doctor, who referred him to the local hospital where a compression ultrasound test showed extensive deep vein thrombosis extending into his thigh vein. Bob was offered the options of either being admitted to hospital for treatment or of receiving treatment out of hospital. He decided on the latter course and was injected with an LMWH and started on oral warfarin. He was instructed in the technique of self-injection, counseled on diet and other drug use while taking warfarin, and asked to come back to have his INR performed daily. He had no difficulty injecting himself with the LMWH once daily, and after six days his INR was 2.4 (the target being 2.0 to 3.0). At this time the LMWH injections were discontinued and he continued on warfarin therapy for about six months. He was instructed about INR monitoring, told to eat a normal diet, and encouraged to remain active. He was also told that a decision to continue or stop the warfarin would be made after six months of treatment.

Patients with vein clots are treated with a combination of an injectable and an oral blood thinner. The person is usually offered home treatment with an LMWH. The injections can be given by the patient, a partner, and in some situations, a visiting nurse.

For clots in the deep veins of the legs, immediate treatment is an injectable blood thinner—either heparin, LMWH, or fondaparinux—to prevent growth of the clot or the development of lung embolism. These injectable blood thinners are started straightaway, sometimes even before all of the diagnostic investigations are complete (if, for some reason, the tests are delayed). Treatment with the injectable blood thinner is continued for about five to seven days, along with oral therapy with warfarin. As discussed in the previous section on drugs, the blood thinners—heparin, LMWH, fondaparinux, and warfarin—stop the clot from growing by "switching off" the clot-forming process and allowing the clot to be slowly dissolved by the body's natural defence mechanisms. The dose you take is adjusted according to weight. Heparin requires blood testing with the APTT and dose adjustment based on the result of the test. LMWH and fondaparinux do not require blood testing for dose adjustment; rather, a fixed dose of these drugs is taken based on the person's weight.

Most patients with venous clots—and many with lung emboli—are treated with a once-daily injection of LMWH. In scientific studies this approach is more convenient and has proven at least as effective and slightly safer than heparin. LMWH is easier to use than heparin because it does not require the same frequent blood testing and is taken once daily.

The recently introduced fondaparinux has the same advantages as LMWH. Doctors now teach patients to inject themselves with LMWH. Patients' partners may also perform the injection. Using heparin requires that the patient be treated in hospital, because it is given by intravenous infusion. By using self-injected LMWH instead, hospital admission can be avoided for more than 80 percent of those with venous clots.

Although the thought of giving yourself an injection might seem unattractive and difficult, most people learn how to do it quite easily, and prefer treating themselves with injections at home to being admitted to and staying in the hospital. The risks of LMWH are limited to bruising at the sites of injection. Troublesome bruising can be minimized by learning correct techniques for subcutaneous injection.

The doctor's decision about who will be treated in the hospital and who will treat themselves at home is based on well-established treatment guidelines. If a person is stable, without an increased risk of bleeding, and is able to inject at home, he or she is usually treated at home.

As discussed in the section on blood thinners, intravenous heparin is still used in some patients with lung emboli, but for most venous clots, more and more physicians are switching to LMWH or fondaparinux, also given once daily. Clinical trials have shown that fondaparinux is as effective and safe as LMWH. Fondaparinux is approved by American and Canadian authorities for the treatment of venous clots and lung emboli. It is an effective and safe alternative to LMWH.

In some special circumstances, an attempt is made to dissolve the clot rapidly by using the clot-busting drugs. For vein clots, clot-busting drugs are sometimes used when the clot is fresh and very large, and the leg very swollen. However, as already mentioned, bleeding is more common with clot busters than blood thinners. Anticoagulants are used in 99 percent of leg clot cases. Clot busters are much more effective at dissolving fresh clots than those that are more than two or three days old. Since most vein clots have been present for several days or even weeks before they produce symptoms that require medical attention, clot-buster therapy is not appropriate for most clots. In contrast, most lung emboli arise from fresh clots that break off and produce immediate and obvious symptoms. Therefore, clot-buster drugs are more effective at dissolving pulmonary emboli than they are at dissolving venous clots.

Oral therapy with warfarin is begun at the same time as the heparin or LMWH or fondaparinux because it will be the drug that is eventually used for long-term treatment. Since it takes five days for the full effects of warfarin to kick in, the two drugs are begun simultaneously and the heparin (or LMWH) or fondaparinux is stopped after six or seven days.

How long you will have to take warfarin after an episode of deep vein clotting depends on the nature or severity of the event, the risk of bleeding, and your preferences. Treatment is usually prescribed for a minimum of several months.

Pulmonary (Lung) Embolism

In most cases, the treatment for pulmonary embolism, or clots in the lungs, is similar to that for clots in the legs. It begins with heparin and, in a growing number of cases, LMWH, followed by warfarin in the long term. When treated in this way most lung emboli dissolve slowly and leave no scars on the lung. However, if the lung embolism is very large and thought to be life threatening, it is not advisable to wait for the body to dissolve the emboli slowly. In these cases, clot-busting (fibrinolytic) drugs are used to produce a more rapid dissolution of the embolism.

Fortunately, most pulmonary emboli are not life threatening and in most cases are treated with heparin or LMWH. For those who are treated with blood thinners rather than clot busters, the extra risk of bleeding from clot busters is not worth the risk, particularly as patients respond well and make a complete recovery on blood thinners.

Clot busters can be life saving and should be used if the pulmonary embolism is very large, and therefore, potentially lethal. Potentially lethal emboli are those that are large enough to seriously block blood flow to the lungs. When that happens, the blood pressure can fall to dangerously low levels, a condition called *shock*, or the heart can fail to pump blood adequately, or the blood flow to the lungs is reduced to the extent that the blood cannot extract enough oxygen from the air. Under these circumstances, clot busters can be life saving.

In a minority of those treated with blood thinners, emboli are not removed by natural processes, and a very small percentage (less than 1 percent) will go on to develop pulmonary hypertension or high blood pressure in the lungs. In people who develop this condition, the persisting lung emboli are large and block the blood flow from the heart to the lungs, placing a constant strain on the heart. In these cases, the clot might be removed surgically, a procedure called *pulmonary embolectomy*.

Treatments Effective in Both Deep Vein Thrombosis and Pulmonary Embolism

In both the case of deep vein thrombosis in the legs and pulmonary embolism in the lungs, treatment with any one of these injectable anticoagulants followed by warfarin has proven very effective. Very few patients with either of these conditions—that is, fewer than one in fifty—develop new clots or emboli while they are being treated with these blood thinners. In addition, once treatment with one of these drugs is begun, the likelihood of dying from lung embolism is low.

Blood thinners prevent the development of fatal lung embolism by preventing the vein clot from growing. Most clots that produce symptoms are five to seven days old, become stuck to the vessel wall, and do not usually break off to form lung emboli. However, the older clot can grow and the resulting fresh clots are much more vulnerable to break off and form lung emboli. Even though the blood thinners do not dissolve the older clots, blood thinners do discourage the formation of new, dangerous clots on the surface of these older clots. Blood thinners also prevent the lung emboli from growing within the lungs, and so allowing them to be dissolved by our own natural clot-dissolving enzymes.

Bed Rest and Physical Activities

After a clot is diagnosed, patients are encouraged to remain active. Bed rest is recommended only if it is required because of severe leg pain or, in the case of pulmonary embolism, chest pain or shortness of breath. In our clinics, four out of five people with venous clots or lung embolism are never admitted to hospital. Rather, they are taught to inject themselves with LMWH, are treated at home, and are encouraged to walk around within the limitations of their symptoms. Similarly, people who suffer from leg vein clots or lung emboli and who are treated in hospital should remain as active as their symptoms allow. Typically, for the first few days the patient's symptoms limit activity to walking short distances. In most cases, however, the symptoms ease within three or four days, at which time people are encouraged to gradually return to their normal physical activity. Within a month, patients can cycle, jog, swim, or play tennis or golf. The only activities discouraged are those that could lead to serious bleeding while the person is being treated with blood thinners; activities such as vigorous downhill skiing, extreme mountain biking, and contact sports are discouraged.

Filters

Even if used properly, blood thinners can produce bleeding; as a result, they should not be used by people who already have a very high underlying risk of bleeding. For example, patients who develop a venous clot but also have a bleeding ulcer should not receive this kind of treatment. Similarly, blood thinners might be dangerous to use in people who have recently had a major operation or suffered internal trauma from a motor vehicle accident.

In these people, doctors will sometimes use a filter, inserted into the main vein (called the inferior vena cava), to trap any clots that might break off from clots in the leg and travel back toward the heart. After freezing the skin with a local anesthetic, the filter is inserted through a vein in the neck or groin. It is not difficult to insert.

The development of filters

The history of filter development is interesting. Forty years ago, patients with vein clots who could not be treated with anticoagulants because of a bleeding risk were treated by having a ligature tied around their inferior vena cava. It was soon noticed that this led to serious leg swelling because it produced strong interference with the return of blood from the legs.

Creative surgeons then developed methods of fashioning devices that produced partial tying off of the inferior vena cava, leaving small channels that allowed blood to flow through, while blocking passage of large emboli. These procedures required surgery under general anesthetic.

The next step was to develop metal filters that were inserted into a vein in the groin or neck. Initially, these filters were permanent, but more recently temporary filters have been developed that can be removed if the bleeding risk is only temporary. If a permanent filter is used, doctors will often use blood thinners as soon as the risk of bleeding has subsided. The presence of the filter in the bloodstream can increase the risk of venous clots.

Dorothy, aged 62, had ulcerative colitis (inflammation of the bowel) and was admitted to hospital because of severe bleeding from the bowel. Although confined to bed rest, she did not receive preventative blood thinners (because she was actively bleeding) and on the third day developed right leg pain and swelling. A venous clot was diagnosed by ultrasound.

Dorothy was in a serious situation. Blood thinners could not be used because they might have caused fatal bleeding. Without blood thinners there was a high risk (about 50 percent) that a clot would break off and cause a pulmonary embolism. A permanent filter was inserted because Dorothy's condition was chronic and could return. If Dorothy had developed venous thrombosis one day after major surgery for inflamed gall bladder disease, a temporary filter could have been inserted and then removed after a few days after the risk of serious bleeding with blood thinners was reduced.

Symptom Relief

The symptoms of venous clots are pain, tenderness, and swelling of the leg. The symptoms arise from the continued growth of the clot: as it expands, it causes progressive pooling of blood in the veins of the leg, which in turn leads to swelling and discomfort. The clot also releases chemicals (called enzymes) that cause the surrounding vessel to become inflamed. Blood-thinning medications such as heparin can reduce the production of these pain-promoting enzymes, reducing the inflammation and preventing the clot from growing. Some patients may also require pain medications, but these symptoms usually begin to improve as soon as blood thinners are started and weight is taken off the affected leg.

Blood thinners do relieve the acute symptoms of venous clots, but in about one in three patients, some long-term swelling can remain. Although blood thinners allow natural processes to dissolve most pulmonary emboli, they are not as effective in allowing these processes to dissolve venous clots. As a result, in about 50 percent of patients with venous clots, the clot remains as a scar on the vein and can produce permanent symptoms of pain and swelling.

This long-term swelling, along with the destruction of the tiny valves in the vein, can result in a progressive condition called post-thrombotic syndrome, where pressure builds on the valves below the one originally damaged by the clot, eventually damaging them in turn. Some chronic swelling occurs in about 40 percent of cases, and it can be severe in about 20 percent of cases.

Treatment of Superficial Vein Thrombosis

Superficial vein thrombosis (also referred to as superficial thrombophlebitis) is usually caused by inflammation of the wall of a small, superficial vein. The inflamed vein then acts as a trigger for thrombosis. As discussed, superficial veins are small and easily seen because they are located just under the skin. The superficial thrombosis presents as a red streak that characterizes the clotted inflamed vein.

Superficial clots can complicate varicose veins or occur out of the blue. Sometimes people suffer repeated episodes of superficial thrombophlebitis, but often they occur as single events. Superficial thrombi are usually not dangerous provided that they don't extend into the deep venous system. Uncommonly, they can extend up from the superficial vein (the saphenous vein) that runs along the inside of the thigh into the deep veins in the groin or from a smaller superficial vein into a deep calf vein. In uncomplicated cases, superficial thrombi are treated with anti-inflammatory drugs (for example, acetylsalicylic acid). For stubborn cases that do not subside with anti-inflammatory drugs, blood thinners might be required for a period of two to four weeks. Blood thinners are also required if the superficial clot spreads into the deep venous system.

Treatment of Venous Clots at Other Sites

Venous clots that occur in the arm, brain, kidney, and other sites are treated with blood thinners. Cerebral venous clots are treated for at least six months and sometimes indefinitely. Arm vein clots are treated for three months. Clots in intestinal veins (mesenteric veins) can destroy a segment of the bowel and, if they do, the affected segment has to be removed surgically. Blood thinners might be used after surgery, depending on the cause of the mesenteric vein clot.

In summary, then, most patients with venous clots or lung emboli do very well with treatment. The most serious consequence is death from a large lung embolus, but as we discussed, this outcome is very uncommon if treatment is started promptly and continued for an appropriate period of time.

Avoiding Recurrence

After one episode of venous clotting or pulmonary embolism, it is an important priority to prevent these clots from recurring. A recurrent leg clot, for example, increases the risk that post-thrombotic syndrome will develop, and a recurrent lung embolism could prove to be fatal. This risk though, can be reduced by about 90 percent with the continued use of blood thinners. However, because blood thinners can be inconvenient, limit certain activities, and produce bleeding, anticoagulants are not continued for life in many patients who suffer one episode of venous clotting.

The risk of recurrence when anticoagulant treatment is discontinued varies, depending on the circumstances that led to the initial clot. People at high risk of recurrence when anticoagulants are stopped might choose to continue anticoagulants indefinitely; those at low risk are advised to stop anticoagulants after three to six months, as are those with an unusually high risk of bleeding. Fortunately, it is possible to come up with a reliable estimate of the risk of recurrence in individual patients and provide accurate information of the relative benefits and risks of continuing anticoagulant therapy. Ultimately, the decision to continue or stop anticoagulants is made after the physician discusses the risk of recurrence if anticoagulants are stopped and the risk of bleeding if they are continued.

The following examples illustrate this point.

Bill, age 34, developed a large blood clot in his left leg. He had no obvious risk factors, but his mother and maternal grandfather both had a history of venous thrombosis. He was tested for an inherited thrombophilia and found to have Factor V Leiden, a common but relatively weak risk factor for venous clots. He was treated with LMWH for six days and warfarin for six months. He was a non-professional hockey player who played on a regular basis with a group. Playing hockey was very much a part of his life. He was advised not to play competitive hockey while on anticoagulants, because of the risk of bleeding should he sustain a severe injury. He complied with this advice but was keen to go back to playing hockey as soon as he could.

He was told that his risk of having another event was about one in ten in the first year that he stopped taking anticoagulants and that he had a one in four chance of a recurrence over the next five years. He asked if this risk would be reduced if he continued to take warfarin for another six months and was told that the risk would be reduced while he took anticoagulants, but the risk would return when he stopped. As far as is known, the risk of having a recurrence after stopping anticoagulants remains the same, whether anticoagulant treatment is continued for six months, one year, or two years. Bill also asked about his risk of having a fatal pulmonary embolism if he stopped and was told that only 5 in 100 recurrences are fatal, and that this risk could probably reduced further if he sought medical treatment without delay, should he develop symptoms of recurrence. Bill also asked about his risk of serious bleeding if he remained on anticoagulants and was told that since he did not bleed during the first six months, his risk of a serious bleed was only about 1 in 100.

Armed with this information, Bill decided to stop anticoagulants and assured his physician that he would take preventative anticoagulants if he was exposed to a high-risk situation (such as surgery, immobilization in a leg cast, or serious medical illness). He also assured his physician that he would seek immediate medical advice if he developed symptoms of new leg clot (leg pain or swelling) or lung embolism (shortness of breath or chest pain).

Bill made an informed decision to stop anticoagulants after six months. His decision was reasonable.

Now let's look at a similar scenario with a different twist and different outcome.

John, age 34, developed a large blood clot in his left leg. He had no obvious risk factors, but his mother died of pulmonary embolism and his maternal grandfather had a history of venous thrombosis. He was tested for an inherited thrombophilia and found to have Factor V Leiden, a common but relatively weak risk factor for venous clots. He was treated with LMWH for six days and warfarin for six months.

John was a lawyer whose main recreational physical activities were golf and jogging. He was given the same information as Bill and decided that since he had no difficulty taking warfarin and controlling the INR with a home monitor, he would prefer to stay on warfarin and review his decision on an annual basis. His decision was based on his mother dying of pulmonary embolism and the fact that taking and monitoring warfarin was not a hardship for him.

Presented with the same information, people can make very different decisions based on lifestyle factors and personal preferences. Both Bill's and John's decisions were reasonable.

The decision to stop anticoagulants is much easier if the risk of recurrence is less when treatment is stopped or if the risk of bleeding is high while taking anticoagulants. The following two cases illustrate these points.

Elizabeth, age 44, developed a blood clot in her right leg. Two months earlier she had slipped on the ice and fractured her right leg. The leg was immobilized in a splint. After six weeks she noticed that her leg had become painful. The splint was removed and a compression ultrasound showed that she had a venous clot extending from her calf vein into her thigh vein. She was treated with LMWH for six days and warfarin for six months.

At the time she had recovered completely from the leg fracture and was walking normally. She was told that her risk of having another event was about 3 in 100 within the first year of stopping anticoagulants and that she had less than a one in ten chance of a recurrence over the next five years. She asked about her risk of serious bleeding if she remained on anticoagulants and was told that since she had not bled during the first six months, her risk of a serious bleed was only about 1 in 100. Given this information, Elizabeth was content to heed her doctor's advice to stop taking anticoagulants after six months. She was advised to take preventative anticoagulants if she was exposed to a high-risk situation in the future (surgery, immobilization in a leg cast, or serious medical illness). She also assured her physician that she would seek immediate medical advice if she developed new symptoms of venous clots or lung emboli. She asked about future use of estrogens either for contraception or hormone replacement when she reached menopause. She was told that estrogens would likely increase her risk of recurrence and should be avoided if possible.

The risk of recurrence after stopping anticoagulants is much lower if the initial episode occurs in the context of a temporary risk factor that gets better.

James, age 75, developed a blood clot in his left leg. He had no obvious risk factors and no family history of blood clots. He had high blood pressure, controlled by medication, and had

had a stroke. He was treated with LMWH for six days and warfarin for six months. His INR was difficult to control and he noticed excessive bruising on his arms. Although his risk of recurrence off anticoagulant treatment was about 7 in 100 in the first year after stopping treatment, he was advised to stop. This decision was reached because his history of high blood pressure and stroke placed him at increased risk of a bleed into his brain (cerebral hemorrhage) during anticoagulant therapy.

When continuing anticoagulant therapy increases the risk of serious bleeding, it is reasonable to stop treatment after six months.

Continuing Treatment with Warfarin

In the previous section on immediate treatment, we discussed the usual medical treatment of acute clots. In the past, the initial treatment was always in hospital, with intravenous heparin, whereas now the initial treatment is usually with LMWH, and many people are treated at home. As mentioned, after a six- to seven-day course of injectable blood thinners, treatment is continued with another blood thinner, warfarin or coumadin, that is taken by mouth. Both the injectable blood thinner (heparin, LMWH, or fondaparinux) and warfarin are started at the same time, but while the effect of the injectable drugs is almost immediate, warfarin takes about five days to start working. The injectable blood thinner is continued until it is certain that warfarin is having its full anticoagulant effect.

Continued treatment with warfarin is important, since scientific studies have shown that the first clot remains active and capable of growing for weeks to months and therefore the risk of having a second episode persists for at least three months. The oral blood thinner warfarin is more convenient for patients than the use of an injectable drug. Warfarin is very effective in preventing new clot formation and is continued for a minimum of three months in some people, and longer in others.

For most patients, warfarin is just as effective as injectable LMWH and has the advantage of being effective when taken orally. However, there is one exception, and that is for those people who have cancer and venous clots. For them, LMWH is somewhat more effective than warfarin. Accordingly, some physicians treat these patients with LMWH. However, since warfarin is still very effective, some physicians prefer its convenience. If LMWH is used, patients are taught how to inject themselves once daily and are advised to continue this treatment on a long-term basis until the cancer has been eradicated.

As discussed, warfarin is very effective in most patients with venous clots, but it is not an ideal oral blood thinner because dosage control can be difficult in some people and is influenced by a variety of factors including the patient's diet, his or her overall health, the concurrent use of other drugs, genetic factors, and various other factors.

Maintaining the correct anticoagulant effect of warfarin is critical, because if the blood-thinning effects are too strong, serious bleeding can result. If the blood-thinning effect is not enough, warfarin loses its beneficial effect and clots might reform. The difference between taking too much and too little warfarin can sometimes be small. There is no simple way to predict which dose is best for any given person. The only way to determine dosage is to start giving the warfarin at the average usual dose and test the blood frequently enough to evaluate the strength of the blood-thinning effect. Even after the appropriate dose has been determined, it might change for unaccountable reasons. For example, someone could be in just the right anticoagulant range with 5 mg of warfarin when, for no obvious reason, this dose becomes either excessive (thereby increasing the risk of bleeding) or inadequate (thereby increasing the risk of another clot). For this reason, the dosage of warfarin must be monitored on a regular basis for the duration of treatment.

The INR Test

The test that is used to measure the blood-thinning effect of warfarin is the International Normalized Ratio, or INR. The INR is derived from the Prothrombin Time, or PT. To perform the PT, blood is taken and a reagent, which increases the speed of clotting, is added to the blood. The time taken for the blood to clot is measured. This time (for example, 24 seconds) is compared with the time that it takes normal blood to clot (for example, 12 seconds) and the patient PT is divided by the normal time (24/12 = 2.0) The INR is then calculated by making a mathematical adjustment based on the strength of the reagent used.

People who are not being treated with warfarin have an INR of 1.0 (12 /12 = 1.0). Warfarin treatment raises the INR and, in the example described above, the INR is 24/12 or 2.0. The appropriate or "therapeutic" range that will prevent clotting in patients who have had a previous venous clot is an INR of 2.0 to 3.0, which indicates that the blood is two to three times as thin as the blood of untreated people. At an INR above 4.0 the risk of bleeding is increased; at an INR below 2.0 there is an increased risk of recurrent venous clotting.

The effectiveness of this therapeutic INR range is based on years of experience with warfarin and on carefully performed clinical trials that have shown that with INR in the range of 2.0 to 3.0, the degree of blood thinning is just right. While an INR of less than 2.0 indicates that the blood is not thin enough and the protection against clot growth is incomplete, an INR that is greater than 3.0 indicates that the blood is becoming too thin without providing any further benefit.

The average dose of warfarin to achieve an INR of 2.0 to 3.0 is 4 to 5 mg, but this depends on the patient. The required daily dose can range from 1 mg to over 20 mg. As mentioned, there is no simple way to determine which dose is best for which patient beyond trial and error, because an individual's response has to do with unknown factors that differ from one patient to another. Most physicians start with a dose and check the INR daily. Then, based on the result of the INR after three days, the dose is either increased or decreased. The changes continue until the INR stays at 2.0 to 3.0 for at least two days when the same dose of warfarin is used. A typical example is shown in the accompanying table.

Days of treatment	1	2	3	4	5	6	7	8
Daily warfarin dose	5 mg	5 mg	5 mg	5 mg	5 mg	4 mg	4 mg	4 mg
INR	1.0	1.3	1.6	2.3	2.9	2.7	2.5	2.5
LMWH	90 mg	90 mg	90 mg	90 mg	90 mg	90 mg	90 mg	Nil

Glenda, age 55, developed a venous clot in her right leg. She weighed 60 kilos and was treated with 90 mg of LMWH (1.5 mg/kilo/day) for six days. She was started on a dose of 5 mg of warfarin. On day five it became apparent that the INR would rise above 3.0 if the 5 mg dose was continued. Therefore, the warfarin dose was lowered to 4 mg, which appears to be the appropriate dose for Glenda.

However, even after the correct dose has been established for Glenda, her INR was monitored twice a week for two weeks then weekly, then every two weeks.

Continuing regular monitoring with the INR is required to ensure that the effects of the warfarin dose remained within that therapeutic range on an ongoing basis. In Glenda's case her INR began to fall although she assured her physician that she had not changed her dose. Her dose was increased to 4.5 mg and then to 5 mg per day and her INR returned to 2.5 (see accompanying table).

Weeks of treatment	2	3	4	5	6	7	8	9
Daily warfarin dose	4 mg	4 mg	4 mg	4 mg	4 mg	4.5 mg	5 mg	5 mg
INR	2.6	2.4	2.7	2.6	1.7	1.8	2.5	2.5

Warfarin interference

Factors that can interfere with the effects of warfarin include drugs (some of which can either increase or decrease the effect of warfarin) and foods. In particular, foods rich in vitamin K counteract the effect of warfarin and result in an increase in warfarin dosage requirement. For example:

- green vegetables: lettuce, broccoli, cabbage, spinach
- avocado
- green tea
- herbal medicines

Acetylsalicylic acid and other non-steroidal anti-inflammatory drugs can increase the blood-thinning effects of warfarin, as can many antibiotics.

Why did Glenda's dosage requirements increase? There was no obvious cause, although Glenda's return to her vigorous exercise regimen could have possibly increased her warfarin requirements (an increase in temperature increases the speed with which the body destroys warfarin).

In contrast to Glenda, Robert age 63, had to have his warfarin dose reduced after having had a stable response to a dose of 5 mg per day for more than three months. In this case, Robert developed gastric flu with diarrhea. Diarrhea interferes with the absorption of vitamin K by the bowel and, therefore, since warfarin counteracts the effects of vitamin K, the blood-thinning effect of warfarin is increased and the dose must be decreased.

Although doctors aim for an INR between 2.0 and 3.0, there is some leeway. Some benefit from warfarin is seen with INR levels between 1.5 and 2.0 (although not as much as with an INR of 2.0 to 3.0) and the increase in the risk of bleeding really starts to occur when the INR goes above 4.0. Therefore, occasional INR levels a little below 2.0 or a little above 3.0 can be tolerated. Having said this, every effort should be made to maintain the INR between 2.0 and 3.0, although you should expect that the INR will stray out of this range from time to time.

Used carefully to maintain the INR between 2.0 to 3.0, warfarin is very effective. The risk of developing a second venous clot or lung embolism is very low, about 1 or 2 patients in 100 per year. In contrast, if warfarin treatment is stopped after three months or even longer in certain people with high risk, about one in ten of them develop venous thrombosis in the first year.

However, despite its effectiveness, there is a risk of bleeding with warfarin. The risk of serious bleeding is low—about one in fifty patients per year—provided that the INR is in the range of 2.0 to 3.0.

Fluctuations in the INR are often unavoidable even if you take warfarin properly. The risk of bleeding, for example, is still quite low if the INR climbs to 4.0 but rises substantially at 5.0. Similarly, the risk of clotting is still quite low as long as the INR is above 1.5, but becomes a concern if it falls below that level. So, a therapeutic range of 2.0 to 3.0 allows for quite a large margin of error without placing you at serious risk of either serious bleeding or re-thrombosis. As long as your doctor makes the appropriate dose adjustment promptly, problems are usually avoided.

Typically, monitoring of the INR is performed four or five times in the first week of treatment, and then twice weekly until the correct dose has been established. After that, your physician might gradually decrease blood testing from once per week to once per month, as it becomes clear exactly how much warfarin your body needs.

What is done when an INR is outside the range of 2.0 to 3.0 depends on how far out it is. If it is just outside the range, the weekly dose is adjusted up or down, and the INR test is repeated after one week. If it is above 4.0 or below 1.5, larger changes to the dose are necessary, and the INR has to be repeated more frequently until the dose becomes stable. The dose adjustments are made on the basis of the weekly dose, not the daily dose because there is a delay of two to three days before the effect of a dosage change in warfarin produces an alteration in the INR.

The weekly dose is calculated by adding up the daily dose for a week. For example, if the daily dose is 5 mg per day, then the weekly dose would be 5 times 7, or 35 mg. For a minor adjustment, the dose is increased or decreased by 10 percent to 20 percent. For example, if the INR has drifted up above 3.0, doctors would recommend that the weekly dose be lowered from 35 mg to 30 mg per week.

If the INR is found to be above 4.0 your doctor may ask you to stop warfarin for a day or two, retest the INR and then start again at a lower dose. If the INR is dangerously high, stopping warfarin may not be enough and the doctor may want to use an antidote to warfarin. The antidote is a natural vitamin, known as vitamin K.

While on warfarin, it is important for you to maintain physical fitness and an ideal body weight, and so you are encouraged to remain active both while on the drug and after treatment is stopped. The only restrictions are those activities that are particularly dangerous, since the risk of severe bleeding is increased by warfarin. Obviously, activities like skydiving or playing ice hockey are not recommended for people taking warfarin!

Duration of Warfarin Treatment
Warfarin treatment is given for a minimum of three months after a first episode of venous thrombosis or pulmonary

embolism. But how does the medical profession determine how long you should be treated after that?

The decision about length of treatment with warfarin is based on the balance between the risk of a second clot if treatment were to be stopped and the risk of bleeding if it is continued. People who have a low risk of recurrence when treatment is stopped are treated for a minimum of three months, whereas those considered at high risk of recurrence if treatment is stopped are treated for at least six months. Some patients are treated for life.

An individual's level of risk of recurrence when warfarin is stopped is influenced by two factors: the location of the clot and whether or not there was a reversible cause of the clot.

Location of the clot: In general, patients with calf vein clots have a lower risk of recurrence than those with more extensive leg vein clots.

Presence or absence of reversible risk factor: The risk for recurrence is also determined by the nature of the initial event. Venous clots and lung emboli can be classified as resulting from:

- a major reversible cause such as surgery, trauma, or serious medical illness
- a minor reversible risk factor such as pregnancy, estrogen use, or a long plane flight
- no obvious cause, known as *idiopathic* venous thrombosis
- an ongoing or permanent risk factor, such as an inherited blood disorder (thrombophilia) or cancer

In the context of treatment duration, the term "reversible" refers to whether or not the risk factor is still present at three months, when a decision as to whether or not warfarin should be stopped is considered.

Recent research indicates that in many people with idiopathic thrombosis venous, the risk of venous thrombosis continues indefinitely, in much the same way as inherited thrombophilia. It is likely that many people with idiopathic thrombosis have an as-yet undiscovered blood abnormality. These people are now treated in the same way as those with a detectable blood abnormality.

As already discussed, the recommended duration of anti-coagulant therapy is also influenced by the risk of bleeding when taking anticoagulant treatment and the preference of the person taking the treatment.

If the first episode of thrombosis had a well-defined, precipitating cause—such as surgery, for example—and the cause is no longer present, that person's risk of recurrence is much lower than that of someone who had a venous clot either without an identified cause or with a precipitating factor that does not change, such as the presence of a familial thrombophilia. For those with a strong precipitating factor (such as surgery), the risk for recurrence if warfarin therapy is stopped after the mandatory three months of treatment is about one in thirty in the first year, falling to about one in fifty per year thereafter—provided that the person has returned to normal health and receives adequate preventative care if exposed to a high-risk situation, such as the need for surgery.

The table on page 100 relates the risk of recurrence after three months of warfarin treatment following a first episode of venous thrombosis to whether or not the precipitating factor is known or unknown, or is reversible or irreversible, along with the usual recommended duration of continuing treatment.

Precipitating factor	Level of risk of recurrence after treatment is stopped	Duration of treatment
Reversible precipitating factor (major)		
Surgery	low	3 months
Major trauma	low	3 months
Reversible precipitating factor (minor)		
Pregnancy	moderate	6 months
Estrogen use	moderate	6 months
Airline travel	moderate	6 months
No precipitating factor		
Idiopathic thrombosis*	high	at least 6 months, but indefinite if risk of bleeding is low and patient prefers the safety of continuing anticoagulants
Permanent precipitating factor		
Cancer	high	indefinite
Previous venous thrombosis	high	at least 6 months, but indefinite if risk of bleeding is low and patient prefers the safety of continuing anticoagulants
Hereditary predisposition (familial thrombophilia)	high	at least 6 months, but indefinite, for certain inherited abnormalities (antithrombin deficiency)
Paralysis caused by stroke	high	indefinite
Chronic debilitating illnesses	high	indefinite

* Some, or perhaps many, of these people have an undetected blood disorder.

When clots occur at sites other than the legs and lungs, the treatment is similar. For example, people with clots in the arm veins are typically treated for three to six months, while those clots in the brain or intestine veins are treated with blood thinners for a minimum of six months, and sometimes indefinitely.

Risk of Recurrence When Treatment Is Stopped
Let's now recap the risks of recurrance when treatment is stopped.

Reversible Risk Factors (Major)
In people who develop venous clots after surgery and who are treated with warfarin for three months, the risk of recurrence is about one in thirty in the first year after stopping anticoag-

ulant therapy. Thereafter the risk drops to one in fifty per year. Based on these low risk rates, three months of anticoagulant therapy is usually recommended for such people.

Reversible Risk Factors (Minor)
In people who develop venous clots while taking estrogens, during pregnancy, or soon after a long plane flight, and who are treated with warfarin for six months, the risk of recurrence is about one in twenty in the first year after stopping anticoagulant therapy. Therefore, most people in this category are treated with blood thinners for six months provided that they stop taking estrogens, if that was the precipitating risk factor.

No Precipitating Risk Factor
In people who develop venous clots without obvious cause, the rate of recurrence when blood thinners are stopped is similar and independent of the duration of treatment, provided that treatment with a blood thinner is continued for six months. Put another way, in such people who are treated for six months or twelve months or for two years the risk of recurrence is the same in the first year after stopping treatment—about one in ten. Physicians generally recommend a minimum of six months of anticoagulant therapy and discuss the risks and benefits of continuing anticoagulant therapy indefinitely. Many patients decide in favor of being treated indefinitely.

Permanent Risk Factor
In people who develop venous clots and who have a continuing risk factor, such as cancer or an inherited thrombophilia, and who are treated for six months, the risk of recurrence in the first year after stopping anticoagulant therapy is about one in ten or for some even higher. Many of these patients are treated with anticoagulants indefinitely.

Degree of risk	Duration of treatment	Risk of recurrence when blood thinners are discontinued
major reversible precipitating factor	3 months	1 in 30 patients in the first year (Low)
minor reversible risk factor	6 months	1 in 20 in the first year (moderate)
no precipitating factor	at least 6 months and sometimes indefinitely	1 in 10 patients in the first year (High)
permanent precipitating risk factor	at least 6 months and sometimes indefinitely	1 in 10 patients in the first year (High)

To have a recurrent venous clot or pulmonary embolism is an unpleasant experience because of the pain and discomfort that they can produce. However, the two main reasons to try to avoid recurrences are to prevent fatal pulmonary embolism and to reduce the risk of post-thrombotic syndrome.

You can take comfort in the fact that most recurrences can be readily treated and the risk of dying from pulmonary embolism is low when anticoagulants are stopped. Some people find this low risk acceptable and are keen to stop taking blood thinners as soon as possible.

Most recurrences occur in the first few months of stopping blood thinners; the risk then falls substantially in subsequent years. In other words, if you do not develop recurrence in the first few months after stopping blood thinners, the chance of recurrence is much less in future months and years.

The results of a recent research study that examined the risk of recurrence after stopping blood thinners in a large number of people with idiopathic venous clots (no obvious cause) is summarized in the graph on page 103. This shows that most recurrences occur in the first weeks to months after stopping anticoagulants and if a recurrence has not occurred in the subsequent six months, then the chance of having one is lower and decreases over time. Nevertheless, there is this substantial risk of recurrence in the first few months after stopping anticoagulant therapy.

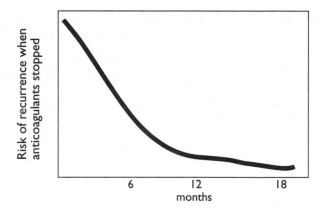

You might ask why treatment is not given indefinitely to all patients who have a high risk of recurrence after blood thinners are stopped. If oral anticoagulants were convenient, safe, and did not have an impact on the quality of life of people who took them, most high-risk patients would be treated for life.

However, the long-term use of oral blood thinners complicates a person's life and is associated with a risk of bleeding. The idea is to balance the risks and inconvenience against the benefits of treatment.

All patients with venous clots or lung emboli should be treated for at least three months, because a shorter course of treatment is associated with a high rate of recurrence. In people with low risk, the risk of dying from a recurrent clot is about 1 in 500 if the warfarin is stopped after the regular period of treatment. In people with high risk, this risk of dying from pulmonary embolism increases to about 1 in 200 per year in the first year after it is stopped, and lowers thereafter.

How does this compare with the risk of a very serious or fatal bleed while on anticoagulants? For the average person the risk of a serious bleed is about 1 in 50 per year and the risk of a fatal bleed is about 1 in 500 per year. Most of the serious non-fatal bleeds have no long-term consequences, but a small number cause permanent brain damage from a bleed into the brain. For people who are at high risk for bleeding, the risk of dying is greater and might be higher than if treatment is stopped.

The good news for those who decide to stay on long-term anticoagulants is that the highest rate of bleeding occurs in the first three months of anticoagulant therapy. This information is provided in graphic form below. This shows that the highest rate of bleeding occurs in the first three months of anticoagulant therapy and then drops considerably. Therefore, if a person at high risk of recurrence has not had a bleed after six months of treatment, his or her chance of having a serious bleeding episode if anticoagulants are continued is less than 1 in 100 per year; the risk of having a fatal bleed is less than 1 in 1,000 per year. The reason many bleeding episodes tend to occur early in the course of anticoagulant therapy is that factors that lead to a high risk of bleeding (for example, the presence of a stomach ulcer) declare themselves early.

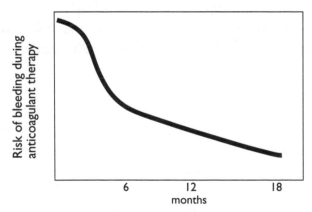

The decision to stop or continue is based on personal preference and the physician's perception of the risks. Based on the foregoing, it might seem that physicians should recommend an indefinite duration of anticoagulant therapy for all those who are classified as high risk for a recurrent event. However, this is not the case, because many people at high risk of recurrance who are faced with the choice of either stopping anticoagulants after six months of treatment or continuing indefinitely make a decision themselves to stop, while the physician recommends that others stop treatment after six months.

Personal Preference

Many people find that treatment with blood thinners restricts their lifestyles; others find it inconvenient and make an informed choice to stop taking blood thinners after six months of treatment. For these people, the decision is a reasonable one. The following are common reasons that people give for wanting to stop anticoagulants as early as they can (which is six months for people with idiopathic venous thrombosis).

1. They cannot participate in their favorite activities; for example, contact sports such as hockey, boxing, wrestling, and alpine skiing.
2. The process of getting blood checked for INR on a regular basis and contacting their physician or a clinic for dosage regulation is tedious. While this inconvenience can be overcome by using home monitors that allow people to perform their own INR reading, these home devices require a certain degree of manual dexterity to operate and are expensive.
3. Some people are uncomfortable with the prospect of taking a drug for a long time, even though there is no evidence that long-term warfarin produces any serious side effects other than bleeding.

Long-term warfarin treatment

If a person at high risk of recurrence who is concerned about the possibility of recurrence of a clot does not find warfarin treatment to be a burden and does not have an unusual risk of bleeding, treatment can be continued indefinitely—or at least until he or she reaches an age (about 70) when the risk of bleeding becomes an important factor.

Physician's Advice

The second reason anticoagulants are not continued beyond six months is because the treating physician advises the patient that, due to a high risk of bleeding, the benefits derived from continuing blood thinners are offset by the high risk of bleeding. As already discussed, the risk of bleeding from blood thinners is greatest during the first few months of anticoagulant treatment and the risk after six months is low in the average person. However, doctors can identify certain people who are at an increased risk of bleeding during anticoagulant therapy. The risk of bleeding, especially bleeding into the brain, increases sharply in people aged 70 (see graph on page 107). The risk is also increased in people who have erratic INR control and in those with a source of potential bleeding (for example, an unhealed stomach ulcer) or elderly people with a history of falling. Physicians usually recommend that people in these groups stop taking anticoagulant after six months.

New Developments

Advances, both in the monitoring of the anticoagulant effect of warfarin and in the developments of new oral blood thinners to replace warfarin, might make the decision to continue treatment more palatable for many. For example, home monitors are now available for monitoring warfarin therapy. These devices are known as point-of-care instruments. The INR is performed on a drop of blood obtained by pricking a finger.

The blood is sucked into a narrow channel in a disposable cartridge. The INR is measured by assessing the movement of blood cells or iron particles. Instruments are small, light-weight, and portable. Point-of-care monitoring has been available in an office or hospital setting for more than ten years. The monitor can be used to control warfarin dosing in the home setting either by people measuring their INR and calling in the results to their physicians—so that warfarin doses can be adjusted (patient self-testing)—or by teaching them to adjust their dosage (patient self-management) based on the INR that they obtain by self-measurement.

Probability of major hemorrhage

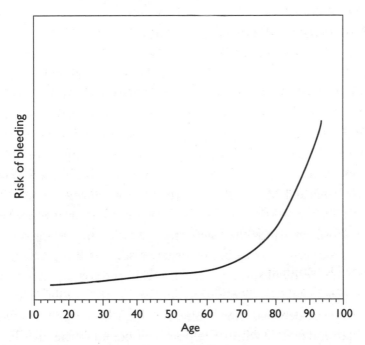

These home monitors are particularly useful for people who travel frequently or who cannot afford the time to attend clinics on a regular basis. Clinical trials have shown that measuring the INR with home monitors is reliable. In some European countries, the patient performs most of the INR monitoring at home. The use of home monitors is less common in North America.

New blood thinners that might not require laboratory monitoring of anticoagulation levels are now being tested in clinical trials. To date, the results have been promising. If they prove to be as effective and safe as warfarin, oral anticoagulation therapy will be simplified, and more people with blood clots might decide to stay on treatment indefinitely.

However, all blood thinners increase the risk of bleeding, and this complication will remain a limitation to indefinite treatment, particularly in those who are at high risk of bleeding, and in those who want to participate in risky activities.

Recognizing Recurrent Clots

Once the decision is made to discontinue treatment with warfarin, there are two things you can do to prevent a recurrent episode. The first is to make sure that you receive adequate prevention when exposed to major risk factors such as surgery, leg trauma, or confinement due to a medical illness. These preventative measures would include the use of any of the four blood thinners that we described earlier in the chapter—low-dose heparin, LMWH, fondaparinux, or warfarin—depending on the nature of the risk exposure. Of these four approaches, low-dose heparin is the least effective following major orthopedic surgery (that is, bone surgeries such as hip fracture or knee replacement surgery), and LMWH and fondaparinux are the most effective. Some surgeons prefer the use of external pneumatic devices. These are knee-high boots or cuffs that inflate and deflate with air to pump blood out of the calf. They are effective and can be used to replace blood thinners as a means to prevent blood clots during and after surgery.

The second thing you can do to prevent serious complications is to be aware of the symptoms of recurrent venous clots and of lung embolism so that you can see your doctor if they occur. The symptoms of recurrent clots are similar to the initial episode: For deep vein clots, *sustained* pain and swelling in the leg and for pulmonary embolism, *sustained* episodes of difficulty in breathing or sharp chest pain that is aggravated by coughing or deep breathing. The term "sustained" is important. Many people who have suffered a blood clot become acutely aware of any aches in their legs or chest. Having said this, the diagnosis of recurrence can be difficult, as evidenced by the fact that fewer than half of the people referred to our clinic with suspected recurrence actually turn out to have recurrent clots. This is because many other medical problems can cause similar symptoms, and because those who have had previous clots (and their physicians) might over-react to minor symptoms that are not caused by recurrent venous clots.

The most common of these "false-alarm" symptoms are fleeting episodes of leg pain or discomfort, chest pain, or difficulty taking a breath. These false symptoms typically last seconds or minutes, and are not the result of venous clots or lung embolism. Constant dull chest pain that lasts for days at a time is another common false symptom of blood clots.

The cause of these false symptoms is unclear. We all get aches and pains, and often think nothing of them. However, quite understandably, people who have suffered venous clots or lung embolism are on the lookout for symptoms of recurrent clots and, when they develop symptoms that they think could be caused by a new episode, they become anxious and the symptoms become magnified in their minds. Some of these fleeting symptoms could even be caused by anxiety and stress.

There are a number of other reasons that the diagnosis of recurrent clots might be difficult. In someone who has post-thrombotic syndrome—that is, pain and swelling from the destruction of venous valves by the previous clot—recurrent venous clots are often suspected when the patient develops more swelling or discomfort than he or she usually experiences. Sometimes there is an obvious cause for the exaggerated symptoms, such as unusual activity, hiking or jogging perhaps, the previous day, but often there is no obvious cause. In this situation, the diagnosis of a new episode of clotting can usually be made or excluded by repeating the venous ultrasound test, particularly if there is a previous test available for comparison.

Similarly, the diagnosis of lung embolism can be sometimes difficult to establish. Occasionally, people who have had an episode of lung embolism complain of recurrent sharp chest pain that is aggravated by breathing, but when they have a lung scan or CT scan, they have no evidence of a new lung embolism. We attribute these symptoms to inflammation of the lung or lung lining (called the pleura) produced by the original embolism. Often, when a recurrent event is excluded as the cause of these various symptoms, the patient is reassured and either has fewer such episodes or is able to cope with the symptoms without undue distress.

Other difficulties in the diagnosis of recurrent venous clots are related to problems in interpreting the results of tests in a person who had a previous episode of venous clots. The problem here is that only about half of all venous clots break up completely. Therefore about one-half of all people with venous clots continue to have an abnormal venous ultrasound test, even years after the first event. If they develop new symptoms in the leg that was initially affected, and the previous venous ultrasound is not available to use as a baseline for comparison, the technician performing the second ultrasound might misinterpret the abnormal result to indicate a new blood clot, when in reality the abnormality is caused by the first venous clot.

Other tests such as the D-dimer or, sometimes, a venogram can be performed to sort out the true diagnosis. A similar problem can occur in diagnosing recurrent lung emboli. For this reason, it is suggested that when people develop new symptoms, they return to the original hospital or clinic that performed the test for the first episode of clotting. Unfortunately, this is not always possible. However, if you have a suspected recurrence, be aware of this potential problem and always tell the examining physician that you had a previous clotting event. The process of making a correct diagnosis of a new clot can also be simplified by having a baseline test performed when anticoagulant treatment is stopped.

In summary, there are several steps you can take to reduce your chances of having a recurrent episode of venous clotting or pulmonary embolism, and to ensure the correct diagnosis is made if you develop new symptoms after you discontinue treatment with warfarin.

- First, you should be given effective prophylactic (preventative) treatment with one of the four drugs we've discussed when you are exposed to *any* of the major transient reversible risk factors for clotting.
- Second, you should remain vigilant to the symptoms of recurrent venous clots and pulmonary embolism, and report to your physician or to the emergency department of a hospital if you develop these symptoms.
- Third, if you develop new symptoms, the diagnostic process is made easier if you have a baseline venous ultrasound, or lung or CT scans performed when anticoagulant therapy is discontinued, so that the results of the baseline and subsequent tests can be compared. This type of comparison,

while ideal, is often not possible. In these cases, the physician must rely on the results of tests performed at the time that new symtoms develop to either make a diagnosis of recurrence or to exclude such a diagnosis.

Treatment of Long-Term Complications

Accurate diagnosis and rapid treatment can prevent many of the long-term complications of venous clots and pulmonary embolism. When long-term complications do develop, what kind of treatments are available to counteract them?

Post-Thrombotic Syndrome

As we discussed earlier, one of the outcomes of clots in the leg veins is damage to the delicate valves that keep blood from flowing backward when we stand up. The quicker the clot is dissolved, the less likely it is that the valves will be damaged. Unfortunately, though, damage can occur before you even know anything is wrong, because vein clots are usually present for several days before they cause any pain or swelling. So even with the best medical care, post-thrombotic syndrome can still occur.

Blood thinners do not dissolve clots; they stop them from growing and allow the body's enzymes to remove them. Doctors have two methods to speed up clot removal. One is to use the clot-busting or fibrinolytic drugs that we discussed earlier in this chapter. The other is to surgically remove the clot. Although both of these approaches are used and are very effective for the treatment of coronary thrombosis, neither is commonly used to treat venous clots because they are not likely to prevent valve damage, and they create greater risks from bleeding than blood thinners do.

Clot-busting drugs, for example, are effective only when the clot is relatively fresh. Although part of the clot is fresh when people go to their doctor with venous thrombosis, a large part of the clot is several days to weeks old and cannot be dissolved. Furthermore, in most cases of post-thrombotic syndrome, the leg swelling occurs because the valves in the veins are damaged, and not because of the persistent blockage of the affected vein by the clot. Therefore, there is no guarantee that leg swelling and discomfort can be prevented by dissolving the clot. Finally, as we discussed earlier, serious bleeding is more common with clot-dissolving drugs than with blood thinners. Therefore, by using them, we could be causing more harm than good.

Surgical removal of the clot is an approach that was taken in the past but is rarely used now, mainly because the clot recurs soon after surgery. Having said that, there are some rare occasions when these treatments might be necessary despite their risks. For example, in cases of very marked blockage, the affected leg can become extremely swollen, take on a dark blue color, and be in danger of developing gangrene. In such rare cases, surgical removal of the clot can save the affected leg.

Other surgeries to repair the venous valves—such as grafting in lengths of veins with intact valves, or creating artificial valves—have been attempted. These have not been effective, because the grafts tend to clot up.

The good news is that often (in about 60 percent of cases), there are no clinical consequences of venous clots, and the affected leg returns to normal. However, persistent symptoms of mild leg swelling, particularly at the end of the day, occur in about 40 percent of people who suffer a venous clot. And some, about 20 percent, will develop the troublesome symptoms of post-thrombotic syndrome.

In many of these patients, the leg swelling and discomfort can be controlled by the use of elasticized compression stockings. By compressing the legs, the stockings counteract the increased venous pressure and reduce swelling. The two most serious complications of the post-thrombotic syndrome are leg ulcers (that usually form just above the ankle) and severe swelling and constant pain and discomfort that interferes with normal daily activities. Fortunately, there are ways in which we can help most people who suffer from these severe complications of the post-thrombotic syndrome.

Leg Ulcers

These ulcers usually occur above the inner ankle where blood flow to the skin is most severely limited. The skin around the shin becomes pigmented, or discolored, because of recurrent small bleeds from the thin-walled veins that are distended due to the increased venous pressure. The tiny, thin-walled veins are prominent, and both the degree of discoloration and number of these tiny veins increase with time. The skin can become dry and itchy. It should be pointed out most people with discoloration do not develop ulcers.

When ulcers do form, they are often precipitated by a mild injury to the area or from an ill-fitting boot. Some develop after an insect bite or from scratching the skin in the area. If the skin is dry and itchy, moisturizing lotions are helpful. The ulcers tend to get infected and, if they do, they are difficult to heal. Every effort should be made to *prevent* leg ulcers. People with leg swelling should wear compression stockings when they are on their feet. The area of skin at risk, which is just above the ankle, should be protected from injury. The need to wear protective work boots can pose a problem because the upper part of the boot can rub against the shin. If that occurs, wrapping padding over the stocking can protect the region around the ankle. The area should be kept clean at all times and dryness should be avoided by using moisturizing cream. If an ulcer forms, it can usually be healed by treating any signs of infection with topical antibiotics, compressing the region with well-fitted stockings that are reinforced with compression sleeves that can be purchased at a pharmacy, and protecting the region from injury. In very difficult cases that do not respond to treatment, a plaster cast is used to temporarily immobilize the affected leg.

Swelling and Pain

The second symptom of severe post-thrombotic syndrome is marked swelling with persistent pain. Typically the symptoms are worse after standing or walking and are, to some extent, relieved by elevating the affected leg. However, for some unfortunate sufferers, the symptoms are so severe—as soon as they stand, the swelling and the feeling of intense pressure from the swelling becomes incapacitating—that they become housebound. These unfortunate people can be helped by using a high-pressure extremity pump, which consists of a sleeve that is applied to the leg and inflated to a pressure that forces the fluid out of the leg. It is used for twenty minutes twice daily (at noon and in the evening), and provides relief for a number of hours, during which time the person can perform tasks such as shopping or walking.

Pulmonary Hypertension

Lung emboli are more easily dissolved by the body's natural clot-dissolving enzymes than are venous clots. In most cases, these emboli are no longer present after three to six months of anticoagulant treatment. This is because pulmonary emboli usually arise from a growing, fresh clot in a leg vein that breaks off and travels to the lungs. These fresh clots are usually susceptible to being dissolved by the body's enzyme system.

However, in some cases of pulmonary embolism, a complication called thromboembolic pulmonary hypertension can arise. As we discussed in Chapter Three, pulmonary hypertension results from the buildup of blood pressure in the arteries of the lung because the unresolved clot packs the pulmonary arteries. The thromboembolic pulmonary hypertension can develop years after the initial pulmonary embolism, or it can occur soon after the first event. If it occurs within weeks or even months of the first event, the pulmonary hypertension can get better with clot busters or blood thinners. If the pulmonary hypertension develops years after the first event, it usually does not respond to clot busters or blood thinners.

In the past, pulmonary hypertension that did not improve with clot busters or blood thinners was fatal. However, now it can be treated successfully with surgery. The surgical procedure is complicated, very specialized, and performed under cardiopulmonary bypass. There are only a handful of centers in North America capable of performing the operation, but in the hands of the experts at these centers, most people survive.

Living with Venous Thrombosis and Pulmonary Embolism

What might you expect after you recover from the initial episode of venous thrombosis or pulmonary embolism? After an initial course of heparin or LMWH or fondaparinux, you will be treated for at least three months with an oral anticoagulant like warfarin. Once you leave hospital and start becoming physically active you might notice a recurrence of some leg pain and swelling (if you had a deep vein thrombosis) or some breathing difficulty on exertion (if you had a pulmonary embolism). This is to be expected and does not indicate that the clotting process has returned. With time these

---

Coumadin tips

People taking warfarin should:

- remain active (they can play tennis and golf, jog, walk, or work in the garden)
- remember that excessive activity is not harmful
- avoid gaining weight
- maintain fitness

symptoms will improve, but about 40 percent of people who have had venous thrombosis will continue to have some swelling and variable discomfort in the affected leg. In fewer than 1 percent of patients with pulmonary embolism, the shortness of breath does not improve and might become worse.

Warfarin Treatment

During the time that you are treated with warfarin you should remain active: play tennis, golf, jog, or work in the garden. However, you should avoid activities that could lead to serious bleeding. Such activities include aggressive mountain biking, downhill skiing, and contact sports, such as hockey.

Many people are under the misconception that excessive activity could be harmful. Some reduce their level of activity to the point that they gain weight and lose fitness. Some people are so fearful of the clot breaking off that they walk with a limp to protect their affected leg, an approach that is not only unnecessary, but harmful to their health because it can lead to problems with their joints and disable them. I encourage my patients to return to their normal level of physical activity as soon as they are able and to maintain an ideal body weight.

Warfarin treatment requires careful and regular monitoring with INR measurements. Many drugs, including over-the-counter-drugs, some herbal medicines, and other alternative medicines have the potential to interfere with the blood-thinning effect of coumadin. Therefore, if such medications are being used, you should inform your doctor who will have your INR checked more frequently. Acetylsalicylic acid (aspirin) can increase the risk of bleeding without affecting the INR. Unless your doctor tells you to take it while taking warfarin (which is sometimes indicated), you should avoid all acetylsalicylic acid–containing medications. Remember, many over-the-counter medicines contain acetylsalicylic acid, so read the label on *all* medications.

People are sometimes confused about what they can and cannot eat. You should eat a balanced diet. You can eat green vegetables even though they contain vitamin K, as long as you are reasonably consistent in your eating habits. Problems can occur with the INR if you go on a weight reduction diet that is high in vitamin K–containing green vegetables, and then decide to come off the diet. Sometimes people are concerned because they require a large dose of warfarin to keep their INR between 2.0 and 3.0. There is no need for concern because the dosage requirements for warfarin vary quite widely among patients with venous thrombosis or pulmonary embolism and have no relationship to the severity of the thrombosis or the risk of bleeding. It's the INR, not the dose of warfarin, that is important.

Stopping Warfarin

After a variable period—which is often six months, but could be longer—many people discontinue warfarin. The decision to discontinue should be made after you discuss the pros and cons with your doctor.

Some people cannot wait to discontinue warfarin because they find it inconvenient to have INR testing. More commonly, they find that taking a blood thinner limits their lifestyle. Others prefer not to take the chance of a possible second episode of venous clotting and find comfort in remaining on warfarin. The risk of bleeding with warfarin diminishes with time, so if there are no obvious risk factors for bleeding, staying on the drug indefinitely is a reasonable option for people with idiopathic thrombosis (people with no risk factors). However, after the risks and benefits of coming off warfarin are explained, many people opt to discontinue.

Discontinuing warfarin treatment can be a scary time for some, because the slightest twinge in the leg or chest can be mistaken for a new clotting episode. It is important to recognize the symptoms of a new episode of clotting (venous thrombosis or pulmonary embolism) and to differentiate them from the odd aches and pains that we all get from time to time. People who are left with leg swelling after the original deep vein thrombosis (post-thrombotic syndrome) will often notice worsening of symptoms after they have been on their feet all day, and these symptoms can be quite marked after unusually vigorous activity. This worsening of swelling can be mistaken for a new episode of venous clotting. The symptoms of second episodes of clotting are identical with the first episode, described in detail earlier. In brief, symptoms of deep vein thrombosis are sustained pain and/or swelling of the leg that lasts for hours or days, not minutes. The symptoms of pulmonary embolism are sustained sharp chest pain aggravated by breathing, and difficulty in breathing. The mind can play strange tricks on us. It is not unusual to have people tell me that they have difficulty in taking a breath, or that they get twinges in the chest that last for seconds or a few minutes. These are not symptoms of new clotting and once the patient is reassured, the symptoms often disappear or are ignored.

The risk of a further episode of clotting can be reduced by ensuring that prevention, usually with blood thinners, is used whenever you are exposed to a high-risk situation such as surgery or injury to the leg that requires splinting. The risk of thrombosis with long distance flights can be markedly decreased by either wearing support stocking or, in very high-risk people, by injecting yourself with LMWH before you leave for the airport. If the latter method is chosen, you can be taught to inject yourself and take a vial with you for the return flight. If you are still on warfarin, there is no need for further protection. All female patients should be counseled about using estrogen and becoming pregnant.

SEVEN

Inherited Thrombophilia

lthough thrombophilia (an increased tendency for the blood to clot) is referred to throughout this book, this brief chapter is devoted to inherited, or familial, thrombophilia. It is for the benefit of those readers who want to learn more about this specific condition.

The following aspects are discussed: why some people develop thrombophilia; the frequency of inherited thrombophilia; the risk of thrombosis in someone with thrombophilia; the likelihood that an affected person's children and grandchildren will inherit the disorder; the precautions that should be taken if a person has thrombophilia; the treatment of thrombophilia; the safety of estrogens or pregnancy in women with thrombophilia; and the treatment of pregnant women with thrombophilia.

Normally, blood contains *clotting factors* and *anticlotting factors* that balance each other so that bleeding is stopped when a vessel is cut, and excessive clotting does not occur when a vessel is injured or the blood flow in veins slows down. Thrombophilia can be inherited and is the result of a genetic mutation that produces defective anticlotting factors—which, in turn, cause decreased production of the anticlotting protein or production of a protein that does not work properly.

The origins of the term

The term "thrombophilia" was first used in 1965 to describe a Norwegian family that had an increased tendency to venous thrombosis. Thrombophilia is now used to include any condition that is associated with an *increased tendency to venous clotting*. Some physicians use the terms "hypercoagulable state" and "thrombophilia" interchangeably.

Why Some People Develop Thrombophilia

People who inherit a mutant gene from one parent are said to be heterozygous. Those who inherit a mutant gene from each parent are called homozygous. Most people with inherited thrombophilia are heterozygotes and have only one mutant gene. Since, in heterozygotes, a normal gene (for the anticlotting protein) is inherited from the unaffected parent, the defect is only partial, and about 50 percent of the anticlotting protein is normal—which is a sufficient amount to protect heterozygotes from thrombosis in childhood and adolescence, but might not be enough to protect them when they are older.

As explained in Chapter Two, there are five recognized, inherited thrombophilic disorders: antithrombin, protein C, protein S, Factor V Leiden, and prothrombin.

These abnormalities are detected by performing specific blood tests. Children of a parent who is heterozygous for one of these defects have a 50 percent chance of inheriting the abnormality. If, for example, there are four children in the family—and one parent is heterozygous—on average two children will inherit the defect. However, sometimes, by chance, none of the children will inherit the abnormal gene, whereas at other times, one or three or all four children will have the defect. *Children who do not inherit the defect will not pass it on to their children*—in other words these abnormalities do not skip a generation.

In contrast, those who inherit the defect have a 50 percent chance of passing it on to their children. Not all people with inherited thrombophilia have a family history because most do not develop venous clotting. Those who do respond well to blood thinners, such as heparin and warfarin.

Physicians usually suspect the presence of thrombophilia under two circumstances:

1. when a person develops venous thrombosis without obvious cause
2. when there is a family history of venous thrombosis

The likelihood of finding thrombophilia during a blood test is increased if venous thrombosis occurs at a young age, occurs more than once, or is associated with a family history of thrombosis.

Approximately 50 percent of people who develop venous thrombosis and have clinical features consistent with thrombophilia will have an abnormal anticlotting protein detected by blood testing. *The remainder will not have detectable abnormalities* but might well have an as-yet undiscovered defect, while others do not have an inherited abnormality.

The need for testing all those who show an abnormal tendency to clot is controversial. Some experts advocate against routine blood testing, because it does not influence treatment. Instead, these experts recommend the same duration of treatment if a clot develops—regardless of whether or not a blood defect is found. This approach is very reasonable for the treatment of patients who present with thrombosis.

However, many patients want to know whether they have a defect and, more importantly, whether it has been passed on to their children. Moreover, it is especially important to know whether a female child has inherited the abnormality since such knowledge could influence the decision about the use of birth control pills or the management of pregnancy. This is discussed in more detail later.

The Frequency of Inherited Thrombophilia

Thrombophilic abnormalities are common in the normal population and most people who have them do not develop clotting problems. Therefore, if an abnormality is found on routine blood testing, there is no cause for concern as such defects are more common in those who develop unprovoked thrombosis.

If testing is performed in people without a personal history of thrombosis, an inherited thrombophilic disorder is found in about 8 percent. About 5 percent have the Factor V Leiden mutation, 2 percent have the prothrombin mutation, and the remaining 1 percent is made up of deficiencies of antithrombin, protein C, or protein S. The frequency of Factor V Leiden and the prothrombin mutation is much lower in people of African and Asian descent than in those of European descent. As already mentioned, the frequency of inherited thrombophilia in people with unprovoked venous thrombosis is much higher (about 50 percent). Most of these people have a Factor V Leiden mutation.

The Risk of Thrombosis in Someone with Thrombophilia
Testing for inherited thrombophilia is usually performed in one of two situations:

1. In people who are at risk of being asymptomatic carriers of a mutation. These are asymptomatic people without a history of thrombosis who are tested because one or more family members have an inherited thrombophilic abnormality.
2. In those who develop thrombosis without a major provocation.

Although the risk of thrombosis in asymptomatic carriers is higher than it is in the normal population, it is still quite low. For example, the annual risk of venous thrombosis in a 25-year-old without thrombophilia is approximately 1 in 10,000. This annual risk is increased to about 1 in 5,000 with a prothrombin mutation, 1 in 2,000 with a Factor V Leiden mutation, and about 1 in 1,000 with the other abnormalities.

The baseline risk of thrombosis increases with age. By the age of 60, the annual risk of thrombosis in a person without thrombophilia is about 1 in 1,000, whereas the annual risk in an asymptomatic carrier of the Factor V Leiden mutation is 1 in 200. Based on these figures, most asymptomatic carriers never develop venous thrombosis.

What about the risk of another venous clot presenting in those with thrombophilia who have had an episode of thrombosis? The risk is very low, provided that they remain on anticoagulant treatment. While the risk is higher when they cease treatment, it is about the same as for those with unprovoked thrombosis who do not have an identified inherited thrombophilia. Thus, the risk of developing a second venous clot when someone with unprovoked thrombosis (with or without inherited thrombophilia) stops anticoagulant treatment is about 10 percent in the first year after stopping and about 5 percent per year thereafter. Based on this level of risk, some people prefer to remain on anticoagulants indefinitely and some prefer to stop after six to twelve months.

What Are the Chances of Passing on the Disorder?

If one parent is a heterozygote for a particular abnormality (the usual situation) then on average, each child has a 50 percent chance of inheriting the abnormality. If a person is found not to be a carrier, he or she will not pass the defect on to their children. The need for thrombophilia testing of family members is controversial, and testing should be performed only if the result will influence a family member's treatment.

What Precautions Should Be Taken?

Three different scenarios need to be discussed: the asymptomatic carrier, the carrier with a history of thrombosis who is being treated with anticoagulants over the long term, and the carrier with a history of thrombosis who has discontinued anticoagulants.

1. **Asymptomatic carriers** do not require life-long anticoagulant treatment because the risk and inconvenience of this treatment far outweighs the risk of thrombosis. *Women should avoid estrogen use unless absolutely necessary.* Treatment (usually with anticoagulants) should be used in high-risk situations, such as surgical procedures or immobilization because of injury or serious illness. Precautions should also be considered during long flights.
2. **Carriers with a history of thrombosis who are being treated with anticoagulants over the long term** are well protected and can travel without fear. If they require surgery, warfarin will be stopped five days before and replaced with LMWH (by injection under the skin). This will be stopped 12 to 24 hours before surgery. Warfarin and LMWH is then restarted about 12 hours after surgery. Most physicians advise treatment with high doses of LMWH before surgery and with lower prophylactic doses of LMWH after surgery.
3. **Carriers with a history of thrombosis who have discontinued anticoagulants** should undergo the same precautions as described for asymptomatic carriers.

The Treatment of Thrombophilia

Asymptomatic carriers require treatment only when in high-risk situations. Patients with inherited thrombophilia who suffer an episode of venous thrombosis are treated with anticoagulants for a minimum of six months. If the episode of thrombosis is unprovoked, many will be treated with anticoagulants indefinitely (for many years to life). The decision to either stop or continue anticoagulant treatment is based on the patient's preferences, the risk of bleeding while on anticoagulants, and the type of inherited thrombophilia.

Estrogen, Pregnancy, and Thrombophilia

Estrogens, whether used as contraceptives or for hormone replacement, increase the risk of thrombosis about three- to fourfold. Therefore, unless they are considered to be necessary for quality of life, it is recommended that they not be used. For post-menopausal women with severe symptoms that have not responded to other measures, doctors will sometimes combine hormone replacement with anticoagulants for six months, at which time the estrogen dose is gradually reduced and the patient is reassessed. However, in most cases, estrogen use is avoided.

A question frequently asked by women with inherited thrombophilia is, "Can I become pregnant?" The short answer is, "Yes, you can." Although it has been suggested that women with thrombophilia have a higher than normal risk of miscarriage, recent evidence suggests that the rate of miscarriage is not much different than in women without thrombophilia. The potential problems with pregnancy are:

- Women with inherited thrombophilia have an increased risk of venous thrombosis during pregnancy and in the first few months after delivery.
- The use of anticoagulants is not straightforward in pregnancy.

The risk of thrombosis appears to be higher in women with antithrombin deficiency than with other forms of inherited thrombophilia, as well as those who have had a previous episode of thrombosis. The use of anticoagulants in pregnancy is not straightforward because warfarin crosses the placenta and can produce defects in the unborn baby (fetus). Heparin and LMWH are safe for the fetus, but heparin can cause bone loss in the mother. Therefore, when anticoagulants are required during pregnancy, LMWH is used. It must be given by subcutaneous injection, usually one injection per day. The patient or a partner is taught how to inject the medication at home. Warfarin can be used after delivery, even in women who breast-feed, so the use of anticoagulants is not a problem *after* delivery.

A number of approaches can be used for women with thrombophilia who are pregnant or desire to become pregnant. The choice is based on the degree of risk of thrombosis and on a patient's preferences. The approaches include:

- doing nothing more than careful clinical monitoring for venous clots
- using anticoagulants after delivery for six weeks to three months
- using LMWH for the duration of the pregnancy, switching to warfarin after delivery

If women with thrombophilia develop venous thrombosis during pregnancy, doctors will prescribe LMWH during pregnancy and warfarin after delivery.

Finally, if a woman with thrombophilia who is being treated with warfarin for a previous episode of venous thrombosis wants to become pregnant, doctors can either replace the warfarin with LMWH (when conception is planned) or perform twice-weekly pregnancy tests and stop warfarin as soon as pregnancy is diagnosed.

These management decisions are complicated and need to be discussed with a physician who specializes in venous thrombosis.

EIGHT

Thrombosis in Children

Although venous clots are very uncommon in children, they can occur. Indeed, about 1 in every 100,000 children will develop a blood clot; 5 in every 10,000 children admitted to hospital suffer from a blood clot. The occurrence of clots in children is very trying for the parents as well as the child. Learning about these clots and their treatment helps both patient and parents to cope.

Most children diagnosed with venous clots have an associated illness or condition, such as cancer, major trauma or surgery, treatment with chronic total parenteral nutrition (TPN), systemic lupus erythematosus (SLE), severe kidney disease, or congenital heart disease. Venous clots can also complicate a premature birth.

An important feature that distinguishes between venous thrombosis in children and adults is the location of blood clots. More than 50 percent of clots in childhood occur in the veins draining the arms. This is in contrast to adults where more than 95 percent of clots develop in the veins draining the legs. Rarely, children can develop blood clots in veins draining the kidneys or liver. Although venous clots occur in all age groups of children, teenagers and newborns under the age of 1 are at the highest risk for clotting.

Most clots in children occur as a complication of the use of central venous lines (CVLs), which are used to supply essential nutrients, fluids, and medications to children who cannot take in food or drink by mouth. CVLs can be lifesaving for children who are being treated for serious conditions such as cancer and major trauma. Unfortunately, they can also lead to thrombosis because they cause damage to blood vessel walls, interfere with blood flow in the arm, or contain chemicals (such as chemotherapy) that make blood more prone to clotting.

Similar to those clots found in adults, venous clots that develop in children can break off and travel to the lungs to cause pulmonary embolism, but this complication of venous clots is less likely in children than adults. The other problems caused by arm vein clots is that they can block the CVL and result in the need for repeated CVLs. They can also lead to the appearance of prominent veins on the face and arms. The long-term complications of and problems from venous clots in children are similar to those seen in adults and include recurrent blood clots, dependence on anticoagulants, and post-thrombotic syndrome. However, venous clots are less likely to cause death from embolism in children. As in adults, death and post-thrombotic syndrome can be prevented by following the prescribed anticoagulant therapy program and by wearing below-knee pressurized stockings daily (for leg vein clots) beginning within a few months of diagnosis.

Diagnosis

The symptoms of venous thrombosis in children are similar to those of adults. Symptoms associated with CVL-related thrombosis are subtle and include:

- poor CVL function
- swelling, pain, and discoloration of the affected arm
- swelling of the face and head

- prominent dilated (enlarged) veins on the surface of chest or limb

If pulmonary embolism develops, symptoms could include:

- sudden onset of breathing difficulties
- chest pain that is aggravated by inhalation
- coughing with blood

As in the adult, a suspected diagnosis must be confirmed by special tests. Venograms and linograms are the most accurate radiographic tests used. The use of linograms is specific for CVL-related cases. For this procedure, dye is injected directly into the CVL. Ultrasound can also be used, but this is not as reliable as venograms and linograms for diagnosis of blood clots in veins.

Since pulmonary embolism can have devastating consequences, it is essential that diagnosis is made early and therapy is initiated as soon as possible. Tests used for the diagnosis of pulmonary embolism in children are the same as those used in adults, namely ventilation/perfusion scanning and, if necessary, pulmonary angiography. As in the adult, the D-dimer test (which is performed on blood) is helpful to rule out venous clots and lung emboli.

Inherited Blood-Clotting Disorders

Venous clots can be caused by the same inherited blood-clotting disorder (thrombophilia) that causes clotting in adults. However, although these disorders are present at birth, they are usually not complicated by venous clots until the age of 20 or older. However, if both parents suffer from a clotting disorder, and both genetic defects are passed on to the child, clotting can occur at a young age. For example, children with no protein C or protein S (homozygous for the abnormality) might develop a variety of clotting disorders soon after birth.

Treatment

As with adults, treatment in children also involves the use of anticoagulants. Clot-busting drugs might also be used for the treatment of pulmonary embolism. In children with CVL-related thrombosis, the CVL may be removed as a part of the treatment.

The first anticoagulant given to children is heparin or LMWH, usually through a needle placed into an arm vein. The dosage of anticoagulant is adjusted according to the child's body weight. In most cases, warfarin is given to the child after the first five to ten days of heparin or LMWH use. Warfarin is given once a day as a pill, and the first dose is also based on the child's weight. Interestingly, the dosage requirement of warfarin per body weight is higher for younger and smaller children than for older children and adults. As in adults, the subsequent doses are based on the results of International Normalized Ratio (INR). The normal INR value in healthy children is 1.0 to 1.4. While receiving coumadin therapy, the usual target range is 2 to 3. Warfarin in children is continued for up to six months, and in some children it is continued indefinitely.

In order to ensure that warfarin is used safely in children, certain measures must be taken:

- Parents should make sure that experienced medical professionals including a doctor, nurse, and/or pharmacist are responsible for monitoring the child's warfarin use.
- Parents should be informed about the drug and the INR test and be aware that illnesses and certain drugs and foods (discussed in Chapter Five) can interfere with the blood-thinning effect of warfarin.

- Older children should wear MedicAlert bracelets.
- Parents should always carry medical information about their child, particularly if the child is young.
- Parents should make sure that school staff are aware of the child's therapy, and emergency contact information should be available to prepare for any emergencies that might arise in school.
- Parents should keep a record of the current dosage of warfarin, INR values, and dose changes. As the children become older, they can become more involved in their own care by maintaining the record themselves.
- Parents should be aware of activities that may be dangerous to a child taking warfarin.
- Contact sports should be avoided, but children should be encouraged to participate in noncontact sports and live a normal life, within the limitations imposed by warfarin.

In recent years, hospitals have begun to develop specialized anticoagulation clinics that provide care for children who are treated with blood thinners such as LMWH and warfarin. In addition, educational information is offered on a wide range of related topics such as reasons for taking warfarin, early signs of bleeding complications, drug interactions with warfarin, accurate and complete records of warfarin doses and INR values, calendars for recording warfarin doses, and assistance in obtaining MedicAlert bracelets.

In the past, our knowledge of the causes, diagnosis, and treatment of blood clots in children was limited, and parents had difficulty in obtaining information about the management of these clots. Now, the situation has changed and there are a number of specialized clinics throughout the world. Parents can be reassured that with the proper care their child can receive good treatment and live a full life.

Conclusion

W e have come a long way in the management of venous thrombosis and pulmonary embolism, and the future is bright. The use of well-tested prevention methods in high-risk patients (surgical and medical) results in a dramatic reduction in the risk of venous clots and death from pulmonary embolism. We now have accurate, noninvasive tests to confirm or exclude the diagnosis of clots in leg veins and in the lung arteries. Progress in imaging tests continues in leaps and bounds, and these tests will become even more accurate in the future.

Treatment is highly effective and the vast majority of patients who develop venous clots survive. For the first time in over fifty years, we have a synthetic alternative to heparin. Fondaparinux is as effective and safe as the heparins.

Despite this progress, not all problems have been solved. We still have only one class of oral anticoagulants—the coumarins (warfarin)—and these remain the mainstay of long-term treatment. Warfarin is very effective, but it requires regular monitoring with a blood test and dosage regulation because the anticoagulant effect of the drug is influenced by illness, diet, and the concomitant use of other drugs. Monitoring of warfarin has been simplified by self-testing devices but remains somewhat tedious. New oral agents that do not require frequent blood testing and dosage adjustment are under development, but none of these drugs has yet been approved for use.

Prevention and treatment of post-thrombotic syndrome is less than perfect. Whether future advances with venous surgical techniques or the use of fibrinolytic (clot-busting) drugs will reduce the frequency of this worrying complication remains to be seen.

Table of Drug Names

Generic name	Some brand names	Action and comments
Heparin	Not applicable	Injectable anticoagulant

LMWH
   Dalteparin
   Enoxaparin
   Tinzaparin*
	
	Fragmin
	Lovenox
	Innohep*
		Injectable anticoagulant

Fondaparinux	Arixtra	Synthetic injectable anticoagulant
Warfarin (a coumarin)	Coumadin	Oral anticoagulant
Tissue plasminogen activator (tPA)	Alteplase	Fibrinolytic drug
Streptokinase	Streptase	Fibrinolytic drug

* *available in Canada but not in the U.S.*

Glossary

Anticoagulants: drugs that are often referred to as "blood thinners"; they slow down the clotting of blood.

Atrium: a heart chamber made up of heart muscle. There are two atria, right and left. The large veins of the body (vena cava) drain into the right atrium and the large veins of the lung (pulmonary veins) drain into the left atrium. Blood from the atria then passes into the ventricles, which are larger and more powerful pumps than the atria.

Arixtra: a new synthetic injectable anticoagulant (blood thinner) that contains the active component of heparin and LMWH. Trade name for fondaparinux.

Aorta: a large artery into which blood is pumped from the left side of the heart and transported to other parts of the body.

Artery: a blood vessel that transports blood away from the heart to various parts (lungs, brain, kidneys, arms, legs) of the body.

Blood vessel: a tube that transports blood throughout the body.

Bronchitis: inflammation of the tubes through which air passes into the lungs.

Capillaries: tiny microscopic blood vessels that connect the arterial and venous circulations. Capillaries in the lungs form a natural barrier that prevents clots that form in the venous circulation from passing into the systemic arterial circulation. Blood flowing in the capillaries provides oxygen and nutrients to the tissues of the body and in turn receives waste products from the tissues that then drain away into the veins.

Calf veins: veins in the leg that are located below the knee.

Carrier: a person who has inherited a clotting defect. Some carriers have thrombosis while other family members do not.

Cerebral artery: an artery supplying blood to the brain.

Compression ultrasound: a diagnostic test for venous thrombosis.

Coronary artery: an artery that supplies blood to the heart.

Coumadin: a trade name for warfarin.

Coumarins: a class of oral anti-coagulants (blood thinners) that counteract the effect of vitamin K (also called vitamin K antagonists). Warfarin is a coumarin.

Dalteparin: a LMWH. The trade name is Fragmin.

D-dimer: a blood test sometimes used to assist in the diagnosis of venous thrombosis and pulmonary embolism.

Deep vein thrombosis (DVT): a blood clot in a deep vein of the leg or pelvis.

Doppler ultrasound: a diagnostic test for venous thrombosis.

Duplex ultrasound: similar to compression ultrasound and doppler ultrasound.

Edema: a buildup of fluid in body tissues that causes swelling.

Embolism: a blood clot that breaks off from its origin in a blood vessel and is carried by the flow of blood and blocks a smaller downstream blood vessel.

Endothelium: the layer of cells lining blood vessels.

Enoxaparin: a LMWH. Trade name Lovenox.

Factor V Leiden: the commonest cause of inherited thrombophilia. It occurs in about 5 percent of North Americans of European descent.

Familial thrombophilia: an increased tendency to clot that is inherited and occurs in families.

Fibrin: a thread-like substance that is derived from blood and makes up part of a clot.

Fibrinolytic drug: a "clot buster" that dissolves blood clots. Examples are TPA and Streptokinase.

Fondaparinux: a new synthetic injectable blood thinner that contains the active component of heparin and LMWH. The trade name is Arixtra.

Fragmin: a LMWH. Trade name for dalteparin.

Heart attack: (also called myocardial infarction) damage to heart muscle caused by lack of oxygen, which usually occurs as a result of blockage of a coronary artery by a blood clot.

Hemostatic plug: a solid mass made up of clumped platelets and fibrin that seals off tears or holes in injured blood vessels, thereby limiting the amount of bleeding.

Heparin: an injectable anticoagulant (blood thinner).

Heparin-induced thrombocytopenia (HIT): an uncommon complication of heparin treatment that can lead to thrombosis or worsening of thrombosis.

Inferior vena cava: A large vein that transports blood to the right atrium from the lower half of the body.

Inherited thrombophilia: same as familial thrombophilia.

International normalized ratio (INR): a blood test that is used to monitor and adjust the dose of warfarin.

Linogram: an X-ray test on a central venous line to detect blockage by a blood clot.

Lovenox: LMWH. Trade name for enoxaparin.

Low-molecular-weight heparin (LMWH): an injectable anticoagulant (blood thinner) prepared by breaking heparin into smaller parts.

Lung scan: a diagnostic test for pulmonary embolism, also referred to as a V/Q scan.

Phlebitis: inflammation of a vein often associated with thrombosis.

Patent foramen ovale: a flaplike opening between the left and right atria of the heart. It is present in the fetus and remains open in about 20 percent of adults. It usually causes no harm, but very rarely provides an opening for venous clots that break off to pass into the arterial circulation and cause a stroke.

Pelvic vein thrombosis: a blood clot in the veins of the pelvis.

Phlebitis: an inflamed vein.

Platelets: small particles in the blood that become sticky when activated to make up part of a clot and hemostatic plug.

Pleura: membranes that line the lung and inside of the chest wall.

Pleural space: the narrow space that separates the two layers of pleural membranes that line the outside of the lungs and the inside of the chest wall.

Pleurisy: inflammation of the pleural membranes. It can cause a sharp pain that is made worse by breathing and coughing.

Pneumonia: infection of the lungs.

Pneumothorax: rupture of an air sac of the lungs that results in air entering the pleural space and sometimes causing collapse of the lung.

Post-thrombotic syndrome: chronic permanent or episodic leg swelling and discomfort that can occur as a complication of venous thrombosis. Typically swelling is relieved by elevating the affected leg and aggravated by prolonged standing or walking.

Prophylaxis: prevention.

Proximal vein thrombosis: a blood clot in the deep veins of the leg that is situated above the knee.

Pulmonary angiogram: an X-ray test to diagnose pulmonary embolism.

Pulmonary arteriogram: same as pulmonary angiogram.

Pulmonary arteries: the blood vessels that carry blood from the right side of the heart to the lungs.

Pulmonary capillaries: tiny microscopic blood vessels situated between pulmonary arteries and pulmonary veins. The pulmonary capillaries release the waste gas, carbon dioxide, into the air sacs where it is exhaled and take up oxygen from the air that we breathe.

Pulmonary circulation: the blood vessels that carry blood from the right ventricle of the heart to the lungs (pulmonary arteries) and bring the blood back to the left atrium of the heart via the pulmonary veins. The pulmonary arteries and veins are separated by capillaries.

Pulmonary embolism: a blood clot that has broken off from its site of origin in a vein and travels to the arteries of the lung.

Pulmonary hypertension: increased blood pressure in the pulmonary arteries.

Risk factors: conditions that increase the chance of a person developing thrombosis.

Spiral computerized tomography: a diagnostic test for patients with suspected pulmonary embolism.

Stroke: damage to the brain caused by a blood clot or embolism that blocks a brain artery (or less commonly a vein). Stroke can also be caused by hemorrhage resulting from rupture of a blood vessel in the brain.

Superficial vein thrombosis: a blood clot in a vein close to the skin. Often called superficial phlebitis.

Systemic circulation: blood from the left ventricle is pumped into the aorta and then passes into smaller arteries that transport blood rich in oxygen and nutrients from the lungs to the organs and tissues of the body. After passing through capillaries and releasing the oxygen and nutrients into the tissues, the blood is transported in veins back to the right atrium of the heart.

Thrombosis: a blood clot.

Thromboembolic pulmonary hypertension: pulmonary hypertension caused by pulmonary emboli that do not break up.

Thrombophilia: an increased tendency to clot.

Vein: a blood vessel that transports blood back to the heart from parts of the body.

Venogram: an X-ray test to diagnose venous thrombosis.

Ventilation perfusion scan: a diagnostic test for patients with suspected pulmonary embolism.

Ventricles: The ventricles (left and right) are muscular heart chambers that pump blood into the aorta (left ventricle) and pulmonary artery (right ventricle).

Venous thrombosis: a blood clot in a vein.

Vitamin K: a vitamin found in green vegetables that counteracts the anticoagulant effect of warfarin.

Viral pleurisy: inflammation of the membranes lining the lungs caused by a viral infection.

VTE: an acronym for venous thromboembolism.

Warfarin: an oral anticoagulant (blood thinner) of the class of drugs known as coumarins. Warfarin counteracts the effect of vitamin K.

Further Resources

U.S.

American Heart Association
National Center
7272 Greenville Ave.
Dallas, TX
75231
1-800-242-8721
www.americanheart.org

American Academy of
Family Physicians
11400 Tomahawk Creek Pkwy.
Leawood, KS
66211-2672
Email: *email@family.doctor.org*
www.familydoctor.org

National Heart, Lung and
Blood Institute
31 Center Dr., MSC 2486
Bethesda, MD
20892
(301) 592-8573
www.nhlbi.nih.gov

Canada

Heart and Stroke Foundation
of Canada
222 Queen St., Suite 1402
Ottawa, ON
K1P 5V9
(613) 569-4361
ww2.heartandstroke.ca

The Thrombosis Interest Group
of Canada (TIGC)
www.tigc.org

Index

A

acetylsalicylic acid (aspirin), 67, 86, 117
activated partial thromboplastin time (APTT), 68–69, 79
advances in treatments, 106–108
age, as risk factor, 19
air travel, long distance, 28–29, 63–64, 101
alcohol during air travel, 28–29
American Academy of Family Physicians, 142
American Heart Association, 142
anemia, 18
angina, 10
angiogram, 57
anti-inflammatory drugs, 86
anticardiolipin antibodies, 24
anticlotting factors, 120
anticoagulant drugs. *See* blood thinners
anticoagulant system, 16
antiphospholipid antibodies, 24
antithrombin, 19, 123
antithrombin deficiency, 22
antithrombotic drugs, 9
aorta, 5–6
APTT (activated partial thromboplastin time), 68–69, 79
arm vein clots, 46–47, 86, 128
arterial clots, 9–11, 10f
arteries, clots in, 1
aspirin (acetylsalicylic acid), 67, 86, 117
asymptomatic carrier, 20, 125
atrium, 5
avoiding recurrence, 87–91

B

balanced diet, 117–118
bed rest, 82–83
bleeding
  and blood thinners, 67, 69, 103–104, 106
  erratic INR control, 106
  potential bleeding sources, 106
  risks of, 61, 62
  and warfarin, 96
blood
  anticlotting factors, 120
  circulation, described, 5–7
  clots, formation of, 7–9
  clotting factors, 120
  coughing up, 39
  hemostatic plug, 7–8
  stagnation of, 16
blood abnormalities
  inherited. *See* inherited thrombophilia
  noninherited, 14, 23–24
blood clots. *See* clots
blood platelets, 7, 9
blood tests
  activated partial thromboplastin time (APTT), 68–69, 79
  D-dimer test, 53, 57–58, 111
  inherited thrombophilia, 121, 122
  INR (International Normalized Ratio) testing, 75, 76, 93–97, 105, 106–107, 131
  self-testing device, 76
  and warfarin, 75
blood thinners
  see also specific blood thinners
  bleeding, risk of, 83, 103–104, 106

cerebral vein clots, 48
deep vein thrombosis, 82
for deep vein thrombosis,
78–80
discontinuation of, and recurrence, 87–89
dosage, 67
effect of treatment, 9
in hospitalized setting, 61–62
injectable anticoagulant,
63–64, 78, 82
in long-distance air travel,
63–64
long-term use of, 103
new oral blood thinners, 106,
108
oral anticoagulant, 73–74
pulmonary embolism, 81, 82
pulmonary hypertension, 116
reasons for discontinuation of,
105
recurrent clotting, 45–46
restriction on lifestyle, 105
side effects, 69, 75
symptom relief, 85
synthetic oral blood thinners,
74
types of, 62, 66–67
bluish discoloration. *See* discoloration of leg
blurred vision, 48, 49
bone density scan, 72
bone thinning, 70, 72
boots, 108
brain
and arterial clots, 10–11
cerebral vein clots, 47–48
breathing difficulties, 32, 38
brown spots, 43
buttock, pain in, 31

C
calf veins, 36
cancer, 17–19, 46, 101
capillaries, 6
car trips, long, 29
central venous lines (CVLs), 129

cerebral vein clots, 47–48, 86
chemotherapy, 17, 46
chest pain, 31–32, 38, 39
children and thrombosis
associated illnesses and conditions, 128
central venous lines (CVLs),
129
diagnosis, 129–131
educational information, 132
inherited thrombophilia,
130–131
location of blood clots, 128
long-term complications,
129
pulmonary embolism, 129
statistics, 128
symptoms, 129–130
treatment, 131–132
chronic illnesses, 27
chronic swelling, 37
circulation of blood
described, 5–7
normal circulation, 6i
pulmonary circulation, 7
systemic circulation, 6, 7
clot busters, 9, 76, 80, 81, 112,
116, 131
clots
see also venous clots
arterial clots, 9–11
in arteries, 1
causes of, 3
described, 9
embolism, 9
formation of, 7–9
hemophilia, 16
hemostatic plug, 7–8
pulmonary embolism. *See*
pulmonary embolism
risk factors. *See* risk factors
stimulation of clot formation,
15–16
thrombin, 15
thrombophilia, 16
treatment of, 9
clotting factors, 120

clover, 74
coffee during air travel, 28–29
Color Doppler, 51–52
complications
    immediate complications, 37
    long-term complications. *See*
        long-term complications
compression stocking, 41–42, 44,
    113, 114
compression ultrasonography,
    51–52, 58
computed tomography (CT) scan,
    57
computerized tomography (CT)
    scan, 48
continuing treatment, 66, 91–100,
    116–118
coronary thrombosis, 112
Coumadin, 74
    see also warfarin
coumarins, 45, 74
    see also warfarin
cuffs, 108
CVL-related thrombosis, 129–130

D
D-dimer test, 53, 57–58, 111
dalteparin, 72
damaged veins, 16
deep vein thrombosis
    see also leg clots
    above the knee, 34, 36
    bed rest, 82–83
    blood thinners, 78–80, 82
    clot busters, 80
    Color Doppler, 51–52
    compression ultrasonography,
        51–52
    D-dimer test, 53
    described, 33–34
    diagnosis, 51–55
    filters, 83–84
    follow-up Doppler, 52
    meaning of, 3
    persistent leg swelling, 40–44
    vs. phlebitis, 34–35
    physical activities, 82–83

    post-thrombotic syndrome,
        40–44
    recurrent clots, symptoms of,
        109
    vs. superficial vein thrombosis,
        35–36
    symptom relief, 85
    symptoms, 35, 36–37
    treatment, 77–81, 82
    venogram, 53–54
    Venous Doppler, 51–52
    X-ray tests, 53
deep veins, 34
diagnosis
    see also tests
    in children, 129–131
    deep vein thrombosis, 51–55
    pulmonary embolism, 55–58
    recurrent clots, 110–111
diet, 117–118
discoloration of leg, 31, 37
discontinuation of treatment
    decision to stop, 104–105
    and inherited thrombophilia,
        125
    and lupus anticoagulant, 24
    personal preferences, 105–108
    physician's advice, 106
    preventative measures, 27
    pulmonary embolism and, 40
    and risk of recurrence, 87–89,
        100–108
    warfarin, discontinuation of,
        98–100, 118–119
drugs for treatment. *See* treatment

E
ear infections, 47
edema, 43
effort thrombosis, 47
elasticized stockings, 61, 63, 113
embolism, 9
endothelium, 7
enoxaparin, 72
erratic INR control, 106
estrogens, 25–26, 48, 101,
    126–127
external pneumatic devices, 108

extremity pump, 115
eyes, clots in, 49

F
Factor V Leiden, 20, 26, 123
fainting, 39
familial thrombophilia. *See* inherited thrombophilia
fibrinolytic agents, 9, 76, 80, 112
filters, 83–84
follow-up Doppler, 52
fondaparinux
    deep vein thrombosis, 78–80
    described, 72–73
    long-distance air travel, 64
    post-orthopedic surgery, 108
    prevention of recurrent clots, 108
    side effects, 75
    subcutaneous injection, 67

G
gangrene, 11
genetics, 19–23
glossary of terms, 136–141
groin, pain in, 31

H
Harvey, William, 3
headache, 47–48
heart
    arterial clots, 10
    described, 5
Heart and Stroke Foundation of Canada, 142
heart attacks, 7, 10, 28, 34
hematologist, 48
hemophilia, 16, 22
hemostatic plug, 7–8
heparin
    children and, 131
    deep vein thrombosis, 78–79
    described, 67–70
    intravenous interjection, 67
    post-orthopedic surgery, 108
    and pregnancy, 126–127
    prevention of recurrent clots, 108
    pulmonary embolism, 81
    side effects, 68–70
heparin-induced thrombocytopenia (HIT), 69–70, 72
heterozygous, 121
high blood pressure in the lungs. *See* pulmonary hypertension
high-pressure extremity pump, 115
home monitors, 106–108
homozygous, 121
hormone replacement therapy, 25
hospitalized patients, and prevention, 60–63
hypercoagulable state. *See* thrombophilia
hypertension, pulmonary, 44–45

I
idiopathic thrombosis, 98–99, 101, 102, 105, 118
immediate complications, 37
immediate treatment, 65, 66
indefinite treatment, 103
indirect blood thinner, 68
inferior vena cava, 83
inflamed vein, 35
inflammation of the lung or lung lining, 110
inflammatory bowel disease, 27
inflatable cuffs, 62
inherited thrombophilia
    antithrombin, 19, 123
    asymptomatic carrier, 125
    blood tests for, 121, 122
    carriers with history of thrombosis, 125
    chances of inheriting, 121–122
    children and, 130–131
    development of, 121–122
    and estrogen use, 25–26
    estrogens, 126–127
    Factor V Leiden mutation, 20, 26, 123
    and female children, 122
    frequency of, 123–125

vs. hemophilia, 22
passing on the disorder, 124
precautions, 124–125
pregnancy, 126–127
protein C, 19, 123
protein S, 20, 123
prothrombin mutation, 20,
  123
recurrent clots, risk of, 124
as risk factor, 19–23
risk of recurrence, 101
screening, 22
thrombosis, risk of, 123–124
treatment of, 125–127
injectable anticoagulant, 63–64,
  78, 82
INR (International Normalized
  Ratio) testing, 75, 76, 93–97,
  105, 106–107, 131
intestines, clots in, 48, 86
intravenous infusion, 67
intravenous (IV) catheters, 46

K
kidneys, clots in, 49, 86
knee, above the, 34, 36

L
large emboli, 38
leg clots
  see also deep vein thrombosis
  arterial clots, 11
  causes of, 11–12
  gangrene, 11
  normal valve function, 12f
  seriousness of, 3–4
leg ulcers, 113, 114
leg vein thrombosis, 34–37
legs, swelling in. See swelling in
  the leg
lifestyle, 116–119
lightheadedness, 39
liver clots, 49
long car trips, 29
long-distance air travel, 28–29,
  63–64, 101

long-term complications
  causes of, 40
  children and thrombosis, 129
  leg ulcers, 114
  main long-term complications,
    40
  post-thrombotic syndrome,
    40–44, 112–114
  pulmonary hypertension,
    44–45
  recurrent clotting, 45–46
  swelling in the leg, persistent,
    40–44, 85
  treatment of, 112–116
low-molecular-weight heparin
  children and, 131–132
  deep vein thrombosis, 78–80
  described, 70–72
  long-distance air travel, 63–64
  post-orthopedic surgery, 108
  and pregnancy, 126–127
  prevention of recurrent clots,
    108
  pulmonary embolism, 81
  side effects, 71–72
  subcutaneous injection, 67
lung embolism. See pulmonary
  embolism
lungs
  arteries of, 6
  clot in. See pulmonary
    embolism
  coughing up blood, 39
  inflammation of, 110
lupus anticoagulant, 24

M
magnetic resonance imaging
  (MRI), 48
McLean, Jay, 68
menopause, 25
miscarriage, 24
mobilization, 61
monitoring, 106–108
movement, to prevent pooling,
  61
myocardial infarction, 7, 10

N
National Heart, Lung and Blood Institute, 142
new developments, 106–108
new oral blood thinners, 106, 108
noninherited blood abnormalities, 14, 23–24
normal circulation, 6i

O
obesity, 28
oral anticoagulant, 73–74
oral contraceptions, 25
osteoporosis, 70

P
pain, 31, 37, 115
paralysis of legs, 27
patent foramen ovale, 34
pentasaccharide, 73
perfusion (Q) scan, 55–57
permanent filters, 84
permanent risk factors, 101–102
persistent leg swelling and discomfort, 40–44, 85, 113, 115
phlebitis, 34–35
physical activities, 117
physician's advice, 106
pleura, 110
pleurisy, 31–32
point-of-care instruments, 106–108
post-operative period, 60
post-thrombotic syndrome, 40–44, 66, 85, 102, 112–114
precipitating factors, 100t, 101
pregnancy, 24, 47, 64, 101, 126–127
prevention
    anticoagulant drugs, 61–62
    blood thinners, 61–62
    effectiveness of, 59
    in high-risk situations, 119
    in hospitalized patients, 60–63
    leg ulcers, 114
    long-distance air travel, 63–64
    movement, to prevent pooling, 61
    outside of hospital setting, 63–64
    during post-operative period, 60
    previous venous clots, 63
    pulmonary embolism, 39
    recurrent clotting, 108, 111
    use of, in high-risk situations, 46
previous history of venous thrombosis, 26–27, 63
prophylaxis. *See* prevention
protective work boots, 114
protein C, 19, 123
protein S, 20, 123
prothrombin, 20, 123
proximal veins, 36
pulmonary angiogram, 57
pulmonary arteries, 6
pulmonary circulation, 7
pulmonary embolism
    anticipation of, 39
    bed rest, 82–83
    blood thinners, 81, 82
    breathing difficulties, 38–39
    causes, 37
    chest pain, 31–32, 39
    and children, 129
    clot busters, 76, 81
    clots in leg veins, 32–33
    compression ultrasonography, 58
    continuing treatment, 116–118
    coughing up blood, 39
    and CVL-related thrombosis, 130
    D-dimer test, 57–58
    described, 11, 38f
    diagnosis, 55–58
    early diagnosis of, 39
    fainting, 39
    fatal, 39, 102
    filters, 83–84
    large emboli, 38
    and leg clots, 37

lightheadedness, 39
living with, 116–119
meaning of, 3
perfusion (Q) scan, 55–57
physical activities, 82–83
prevention, 39
previous venous thrombosis, 40
pulmonary angiogram, 57
pulmonary hypertension, 44–45, 82, 115–116
recurrent clots, symptoms of, 109
seriousness of, 33
severe form, 39
shock, 81
small emboli, 38
spiral computed tomography (CT) scan, 57
symptom relief, 85
symptoms, 31–32, 38–39, 119
treatment, 81–82
ventilation (V) scan, 55–57
pulmonary hypertension, 44–45, 82, 115–116

Q
Q scan, 55–57

R
radiotherapy, 17
recurrent clots
avoiding recurrence, 87–91
cerebral venous clotting, 48
diagnosis, 110–111
discontinuation of warfarin, 98–100
"false-alarm" symptoms, 109
increase of risk of, 26–27
and indefinite treatment, 103
and inherited thrombophilia, 124
as long-term complication, 45–46
major reversible risk factor, 100–101
minor reversible risk factor, 101

permanent risk factors, 101–102
precipitating factors, 100t, 101
prevention, 108, 111
recognizing, 108–111, 118–119
risk of recurrence, 100–108
symptoms, 109
timing of, 102
unpleasantness of, 102
red discoloration. *See* discoloration of leg
repetitive activities, 46–47
resources, 142
reteplase, 76
reversible risk factors, 98–99, 100–101
risk factors
age, 19
arm vein clots, 46–47
blood abnormalities, noninherited, 14, 23–24
cancer, 17–19
chronic illnesses, 27
common risk factors, 14–16, 18
developing countries, 13–14
estrogens, 25–26
inherited thrombophilia, 19–23
intravenous (IV) catheters, 46
long distance air travel, 28–29
major surgery, 15, 16–17
major trauma, 16–17
obesity, 28
paralysis of legs, 27
permanent risk factors, 101–102
precipitating factors, 100t, 101
previous venous thrombosis, 26–27
reversible risk factors, 98–99
and risk of recurrence, 100–101
smoking, 28
stimulation of clot formation, 15–16
varicose veins, 27

S
screening, 22
self-testing device (blood testing), 76
septum, 5
shallow breaths, 32
shock, 81
shortness of breath, 32
side effects
    blood thinners, 69, 75
    clot busters (fibrinolytic drugs), 76
    fondaparinux, 75
    heparin, 68–70
    low-molecular-weight heparin, 71–72
    warfarin, 75
skin ulcers, 43–44
small emboli, 38
smoking, 28
spinal cord injuries, 27
spiral computed tomography (CT) scan, 57
streptokinase, 76
strokes, 7, 10–11, 27, 34, 47–48
subcutaneous injection, 67–68, 71, 73
superficial thrombophlebitis, 85–86
superficial vein thrombosis, 35–36, 85–86
superficial veins, 33, 34
surgery, 15, 16–17, 60, 100
surgical removal of clot, 112, 113
sustained symptoms, 109
swelling in the leg, 31, 37, 40–44, 85, 113, 115, 119
symptoms
    cerebral vein clots, 47–48
    chest pain, 31–32, 38, 39
    coughing up blood, 39
    CVL-related thrombosis, 129–130
    deep vein thrombosis, 35, 36–37
    discoloration of leg, 31, 37
    eyes, clots in, 49
    fainting, 39
    "false-alarm" symptoms, 109
    intestines, clots in, 48
    kidneys, clots in, 49
    lightheadedness, 39
    liver clots, 49
    pain, 31, 37, 115
    pulmonary embolism, 31–32, 38–39, 119
    pulmonary hypertension, 44–45
    recurrent clotting, 109
    relief of, 85
    shortness of breath, 32, 38
    superficial vein clots, 36
    sustained symptoms, 109
    swelling in the leg, 31, 37, 113
    venous thrombosis, 30–34
synthetic oral blood thinners, 74
systemic circulation, 6, 7
systemic lupus erythematosus (SLE), 24

T
tenectaplase, 76
tests
    activated partial thromboplastin time (APTT), 68–69
    bone density scan, 72
    Color Doppler, 51–52
    compression ultrasonography, 51–52, 58
    D-dimer test, 53, 57–58, 111
    follow-up Doppler, 52
    INR (International Normalized Ratio) testing, 75, 76
    interpretation of, in recurrent clotting, 110–111
    perfusion (Q) scan, 55–57
    pulmonary angiogram, 57
    spiral computed tomography (CT) scan, 57
    venogram, 53–54, 111
    Venous Doppler, 51–52
    ventilation (V) scan, 55–57
    X-ray tests, 53
therapeutic index, 75

thrombin, 15
thromboembolic pulmonary
   hypertension. *See* pulmonary
   hypertension
thrombophilia, 16, 121
   see also inherited thrombophilia
thrombosis
   see also venous clots
   meaning of, 9
   and systemic lupus erythemato-
      sus (SLE), 24
Thrombosis Interest Group of
   Canada, 142
tinzaparin, 72
tissue-plasminogen activator
   (tPA), 76
trauma, 16–17
treatment
   avoiding recurrence, 87–91
   bed rest, 82–83
   blood thinners, 66–76, 82
   children and thrombosis,
      131–132
   clot busters (fibrinolytic drugs),
      76
   continuing treatment, 66,
      91–100, 116–118
   continuing treatment objec-
      tives, 66
   deep vein thrombosis, 77–81,
      82
   discontinuation of. *See* discon-
      tinuation of treatment
   drug names, table of, 135t
   drugs used (chart), 77t
   filters, 83–84
   fondaparinux, 72–73
   heparin, 67–70
   immediate treatment, 66
   immediate treatment objec-
      tives, 65
   indefinite treatment, 103
   inherited thrombophilia,
      125–127
   leg ulcers, 114
   long-term complications,
      112–116

low-molecular-weight heparin,
      70–72
   pain, 115
   physical activities, 82–83
   post-thrombotic syndrome,
      112–114
   pulmonary embolism, 81–82
   pulmonary hypertension,
      115–116
   superficial vein thrombosis,
      85–86
   symptom relief, 85
   venous clots at other sites,
      86–87
   warfarin, 73–76, 91–100

U
ulcers
   leg ulcers, 113, 114
   on skin, 43–44
ultrasonography, 38
unstable angina, 10

V
V scan, 55–57
varicose veins, 27
venogram, 53–54, 111
venous clots
   see also deep vein thrombosis;
      venous thrombosis
   arm vein clots, 46–47
   cancer, undetected, 17–18
   causes of, 11–12
   cerebral vein clots, 47–48
   damaged veins, 16
   described, 11–12
   diagnosis. *See* diagnosis
   discontinuation of treatment.
      See discontinuation of
      treatment
   eyes, 49
   formation, 8f
   heart attack, risk of, 7, 34
   immediate complications, 37
   intestines, 48
   kidneys, 49
   liver clots, 49
   living with, 116–119

long-term complications. *See* long-term complications
at other sites, 33–34, 46–49, 86–87
patent foramen ovale, 34
risk factors. *See* risk factors
seriousness of, 33
size of, 33
stagnation of blood, 16
statistics, 13–14
strokes, risk of, 7, 34
superficial veins and, 33, 85–86
surgical removal of, 112, 113
symptoms. *See* symptoms
tests. *See* tests
Venous Doppler, 51–52
venous thrombosis
  see also venous clots
  causes of, 3
  continuing treatment, 116–118
  living with, 116–119
  meaning of, 3
  previous history of, 26–27, 63
  symptoms, 30–34
ventilation (V) scan, 55–57
ventricles, 5
vision, blurring of, 48, 49
vitamin K, 118
vitamin K antagonists, 74

W
warfarin
  and acetylsalicylic acid (aspirin), 117
  after delivery, 127
  average dose, 93–94
  bleeding, risk of, 96
  children and, 131–132
  continuing treatment with, 91–100
  deep vein thrombosis, 80–81
  described, 73–76
  and diet, 117–118
  disadvantages, 74–76
  discontinuation, 98–100, 118–119
  dosage, 92
  duration of treatment, 97–100
  effectiveness of, 91–92
  importance of continued treatment, 91–92
  INR test, 93–97
  interference with effects of, 95
  large doses, concerns about, 118
  long-distance air travel, 64
  long-term treatment, 106
  monitoring of, 106–108, 117
  narrow therapeutic index, 75
  oral anticoagulant, 67
  physical activities and, 117
  and pregnancy, 126
  prevention of recurrent clots, 108
  tips, 116
  weekly dose, calculation of, 97
  weight reduction diets, 118
weight loss, unexplained, 18
weight reduction diets, 118
women
  antiphospholipid antibodies, 24
  estrogens, as risk factor, 25
  and long-distance air travel, 64
  pregnancy. *See* pregnancy

X
X-ray tests, 53